UNLOCK THE THERAPEUTIC SECRETS OF OLIVE OIL

Terry Lemerond

The purpose of this book is to educate. It is not intended to serve as a replacement for professional medical advice. Any use of the information in this book is at the reader's discretion. This book is sold with the understanding that neither the publisher nor the author has any liability or responsibility for any injury caused or alleged to be caused directly or indirectly by the information contained in this book. While every effort has been made to ensure its accuracy, the book's contents should not be construed as medical advice. To obtain medical advice on your individual health needs, please consult a qualified health care practitioner.

www.TTNPublishing.com

Library of Congress Control Number: 2023916683

Print ISBN: 978-1-952507-52-6
eBook ISBN: 978-1-952507-53-3

Editor: Michele Olson
Design: Tammy Wagner
Formatting: Alt 19 Creative

Printed in the United States of America

This book is dedicated to all the true health seekers in the world.

CONTENTS

INTRODUCTION

Olive oil has a long and storied history. As a staple source of light and food that routinely appeared in ancient Greek homes, it was even called "liquid gold" by Homer, the poet who penned *The Iliad* and *The Odyssey* in the 8th century BC. Four hundred years later, Greek physician Hippocrates dubbed the oil "the great healer" due to its wealth of medicinal properties.

Today, extra virgin olive oil (EVOO) has once again become a valued staple in kitchens throughout the world because of its fruity flavor and high smoke point. But while EVOO is truly culinary gold, it's the oil's health benefits that set it apart.

Although EVOO has gained a healthy halo in the media, most consumers aren't aware that the oil has been the subject of dozens of clinical trials investigating its beneficial impact on the heart, brain, immune system, and more. In fact, researchers are continually uncovering even more health benefits. For instance, modern research and centuries of use confirm olive oil's ability to protect against arthritis, cardiovascular disease, cognitive decline, immune system disorders, type

2 diabetes, and even some types of cancer. Spreading the word about these remarkable benefits is why I wrote this book.

But learning about the many ways EVOO promotes health and longevity is just part of the picture. It's also important to understand the elements that go into making the highest-quality and most beneficial oil, and how to ensure you're buying the best. This is especially important since fraud has become rampant in the olive oil industry. Some experts even claim that as much as 80 percent of oils sold as EVOO in supermarkets are counterfeit! What's more, one recent study of California EVOO conducted at the University of California, Davis, reported that a large percentage of the oils researchers tested were of poor quality. More specifically, many of the samples that were evaluated had oxidized due to exposure to high temperatures or light. A large number were also adulterated with cheaper refined oils. Making matters even worse, some of the samples were made from damaged or overripe olives, experienced processing flaws, or were stored improperly.

These problems aren't just limited to oils that come from California. Despite being one of the most regulated foods in the world, imported EVOOs have also landed under the microscope, with many questioning both the quality and authenticity of oils coming from countries such as Greece, Italy, Portugal, and Spain. Fortunately, you'll find usable tips for choosing the best—and the most healthful—EVOO in these pages.

Incorporating pure, high-quality EVOO into your daily diet won't just enhance your meals; it will also improve your health. When Hippocrates said, "Let food be thy medicine," he might well have been talking about olive oil.

CHAPTER 1

Olive Oil Through the Ages

Wild olive trees have likely been around since before humans roamed the Earth. According to archaeological evidence, our Neolithic ancestors collected the fruit as early as the 8th century BC. And researchers at the University of Innsbruck in Austria recently discovered olives and wood from olive trees on the Atlantic coast of Morocco dating back to around 100,000 years ago. This suggests that early Homo sapiens used olives for both food and heat during the last ice age.

But olives—and more importantly olive oil—weren't domesticated, cultivated, and cured or pressed until approximately 6,000 years ago in Syria. While some of these early olives were used for human consumption, most were processed to create lamp oil. As a result, olive oil became so valuable that it cost five times more than the finest wines!

Cultivation rapidly spread throughout the Middle East, and later to North Africa and Spain. Olive trees finally reached Greece sometime in the 28th century BC, thanks largely to the Phoenicians. The Greeks then exported the trees to Italy. From there, the cultivation of olives continued to move westward into Sicily, Sardinia, France, Portugal, Algeria, Tunisia, and Morocco. While many of these countries grew olives for fuel, it didn't take long for the Greeks to find a plethora of uses for olive oil that extended far beyond lamp oil. Over time, that knowledge began to move throughout the civilized world.

Fast-forward to the Middle Ages. Olive oil continued to increase in production and importance, primarily in Spain, Italy, and Greece. The greatest expansion of olive oil production occurred after the 1700s when a large number of olive trees were planted to supply the growing city populations throughout Europe. The result was a drop in price and an uptick in olive oil use. But all that changed by the late 19th century thanks to the development of low-cost solvent-extraction techniques for seed oils such as corn and soy. What's more, the dawn of the industrial age brought new technologies for heat and light such as gas and electricity. As a result, the demand for olive oil dropped dramatically until finally regaining popularity again the 1990s. Today, Spain is the largest producer and exporter of olive oil in the world, followed by Italy, Morocco, and Portugal.

One Oil, Many Uses

Since the Neolithic Age, olives and olive oil have played a central role in our evolution. The following is a brief look at the many ways this "liquid gold" has helped mankind survive and thrive throughout the centuries.

Olive Oil Moves to the Kitchen

By the 5th century BC, olive oil had expanded beyond lamps into the kitchen, where it was used to enhance the taste of food. Ancient Romans were so enamored with the oil that a 2021 study of the eruption of Mount Vesuvius (AD 79) discovered large amounts of olive oil preserved in the bones of the volcano's victims. Based on these findings, researchers concluded that the oil made up a significant 12 percent of the Pompeian's diet. Other investigations note that the average Roman consumed 20 liters of olive oil each year, making it the era's most substantial source of dietary fat.

As the Roman Empire grew to include what's now known as Algeria, Egypt, Switzerland, and Great Britain, olive oil became the culinary oil of choice throughout much of the world. But the fall of the Roman Empire caused a significant disruption to trade, decreasing the flow of olive oil from regions of more abundant production to those where little olive oil was made. It was a problem that took centuries to resolve.

Although trade finally picked up between the 11th and 15th centuries, olive oil wasn't considered a necessity. Trade ships were instead loaded with furs, linen, salt, silk, soap, spices, sugar, tin, and wheat. This continued until the dawn of the Renaissance, when Italy became the largest producer and exporter of olive oil in the world. But, because it was so expensive, olive oil was largely reserved for the kitchens and tables of royalty and nobles throughout Europe.

Olive oil remained costly and was considered an exotic and expensive indulgence for many in Europe and the Americas. Instead, most households relied on seed oils like corn and peanut or animal fats like lard for their culinary needs. But fortunately, interest in the Mediterranean diet during the 1990s led professional chefs and home cooks alike to embrace the culinary charms of olive oil. Over the next 20 years, olive oil became so popular that consumption nearly doubled. But, as history shows us, olive oil's benefits aren't just limited to the kitchen.

Olive Oil's Beauty Benefits Throughout History

Not only has olive oil been used for fuel and food over the centuries, it was also routinely used to care for the skin. That's not surprising since the oil boasts skin-friendly antioxidant and anti-inflammatory properties and acts as a natural moisturizer when applied topically. It also boasts the highest SPF of any plant oils. Together, these benefits made olive oil a prized anti-aging treatment, particularly among the rich.

The rich also relied on olive oil to create cosmetics. Well-to-do women in ancient Greece and Egypt would use an eyeliner made with olive oil and charcoal to darken their eyes. This eyeliner was also used to fashion a thick brow, which was very popular at that time among both women and men. The women also brightened their lips and cheeks with a red-colored paste made from red iron oxide, ocher clay, and olive oil mixed with beeswax.

To keep their hair soft and shiny, women would also turn to olive oil. Applied and left on the hair for hours, it acted like a conditioning treatment. As a finishing touch, the women would adorn themselves with perfumes crafted by mixing the oils from fragrant bark, herbs, and flowers with olive oil.

Olive oil was also a popular treatment among athletes, who slathered it over their bodies prior to training for and competing in sports. According to legend, an olive oil rub helped reduce muscle fatigue and soreness by removing lactic acid. But it was also largely part of the ritual of sport as the Greeks ceremoniously rubbed olive oil onto a athletes' skin then scraped it off with the sweat and dust after a competition.

Religion and Rituals

Olive oil has played a key part in religion and sacred rituals around the world for centuries. In Ancient Greece, the oil was used by the Minoans in religious ceremonies on the island of Crete. The Athenians also used olive oil in worship and during funerals. In fact, when people died, olive oil was used to anoint their bodies and prepare them for burial.

Olives and olive oil also play a pivotal role in Christianity and are mentioned over 150 times in the Bible. For instance, the Old Testament claims that, after the Flood, an olive leaf was brought to Noah by a dove, who told him that the flood waters had abated. And in Exodus 27:20, God instructed Moses to "command the Israelites to bring you clear oil of pressed olives for the light so that the lamps may be kept burning."

Olive oil was also important to commerce and trade during biblical times. For instance, Ezekiel 27:17 states that "Judah and the land of Israel, they were your traders; with the wheat of Minnith, cakes, honey, oil, and balm they paid for your merchandise." Clay tablets from the reign of Nebuchadnezzar also listed allocations of olive oil to Jehoiachin, the young king of Judah who was taken prisoner by the Babylonians in 597 BC and lived in exile for the next 37 years.

But perhaps olive oil's most important use in the Bible was for anointing both the living and the dead. In the Old Testament, the oil was used to anoint kings and priests, and during the offering of purification from leprosy. In the New Testament, olive oil was employed to cast out demons and heal the sick. Because the oil was symbolic of the Holy Spirit, it was also applied to the dead in preparation for burial.

While most Christian churches no longer include these practices, olive oil is still used by some branches of Christianity today. The Catholic and Orthodox churches use olive oil for the Oil of Catechumens (used to bless and strengthen those preparing for baptism) and the Oil of the Sick (used to confer the Sacrament of Anointing of the Sick).

Mentioned more than 200 times in the Torah, olive oil is also important in Judaism and was used to anoint the ancient kings of Israel. It was also the oil used to light the menorah during the Israelites exodus from Egypt. Even today, Hanukkah—the eight-day festival of lights—is linked to olive oil. According to Jewish tradition, when the Maccabees recovered the Holy Temple in Jerusalem from the Greeks, they set about rededicating it to God by lighting the menorah. Yet they could find only enough olive oil for one day. Miraculously, however, that small amount of oil burned for eight days.

Islam also reveres olive oil and considers the olive to be a blessed fruit. As with the Bible and the Torah, the Koran refers to olive oil in significant ways, using it as a way of illustrating Allah's own light. The prophet Muhammad also said, "Eat olive oil and massage it over your bodies since it is a holy tree." Olive oil is also used in ruqyah, a recitation of the Koran while seeking refuge, remembrance, and supplication.

Medicine

Perhaps olive oil's most important role throughout history is as a medicine. Indeed, because of its many purported medical uses, it could be considered the world's first functional food. Hippocrates, the renowned Greek physician, listed more than 60 medicinal uses for the oil. These included treating skin diseases, healing wounds and burns, curing heart disease, relieving ear infections, easing digestive problems, and a variety of gynecological issues, including contraception.

Thanks to Hippocrates, the Greeks became pioneers in using olive oil in concoctions and ointments to relieve cramps, treat wounds and burns, and even prevent hair loss. In extreme situations, a patient's entire body was sometimes immersed in olive oil to soothe pain.

Word of olive oil's medicinal properties spread to Rome where Roman emperor Julian's personal physician used olive oil as a base for antiseptic plasters and ointments to soothe pain and heal wounds, cuts, and burns, following the records of the famous Greek doctor Hippocrates. Pliny the Elder, a Roman philosopher, wrote that green olives and their oil are good for the stomach and in particular to protect against seasickness. In his Historia Naturalis, he listed 48 medicines made with olive oil. He also stated that, when mixed with wine, green olives can cure mouth and ear infections.

Olive oil continued to reveal new curative properties during the Middle Ages as it became a well-known remedy for sore throats, cuts, and bruises. It was also used as a base for salves and ointments. The medical monks of the abbeys used preparations containing olive oil to treat burned skin and swellings, as well as different infections. By the time of the Renaissance, jars containing olive oil had become a staple remedy in all pharmacies.

It's popularity as a medicinal remedy continued throughout the 20th century, largely because of olive oil's ability to reduce mucus and relieve inflammation. These properties made it a popular treatment for both gastric and duodenal ulcers, and it was often prescribed as part of a nitrogen-free diet during the treatment of renal failure. Olive oil was also widely used to treat eczema and psoriasis, and to soften ear wax.

While some of these historical uses turned out to be more myth than fact, modern science backs up many of these claims, thanks largely to olive oil's anti-inflammatory and antioxidant properties. Today, olive oil—especially extra virgin olive oil—is valued for both its culinary attributes and its well-documented health benefits.

The Goddess Tree

One of the best-known Greek myths attributes the birth of the first olive tree to the goddess Athena. According to legend, Poseidon (the god of the sea and religion) was competing with Athena (the goddess of wisdom) for the sovereignty of the Greek capital of Athens. The two deities challenged each other on who would offer the most beautiful gift to the people of the city. Poseidon made horses rise from the ground, giving them to the Athenians to help them during their battles. Athena, on the other hand, caused the first olive tree to spring forth from the earth by striking a rock with a spear. Thanks to its fruit, the Athenians could illuminate the night, medicate wounds, and feed the population. Not surprisingly, Zeus—acting as the judge of the challenge—chose the more peaceful element: the olive tree, thus attributing the victory to Athena, who became the goddess of Athens.

CHAPTER 2
What Makes Olive Oil So Darn Healthy?

Take a sip of high-quality extra virgin olive oil. That grassy taste with hints of fresh herbs and fruit, and the slight catch you get in the back of your throat are all signs that the oil is rich in nutritious bioactive compounds. But, while many people know that olive oil—and especially EVOO—is one of just a small handful of healthy oils, most aren't aware of why it's so beneficial for good health. Let's take a closer look at all the health-promoting secrets waiting for you inside that bottle of EVOO.

Free Radical Fighting Compounds

Extra virgin olive oil is rich in antioxidants, which help prevent cellular damage caused by free radicals. Free radicals are oxygen-containing molecules with an uneven number of electrons. Because of this, they can react with other molecules, triggering a chemical chain reaction that causes harmful oxidation in the body. As free radicals accumulate, they damage cells and can play a role in the development of many chronic health conditions. These include arthritis, asthma, atherosclerosis, dementia, some forms of cancer, and type 2 diabetes.

The good news is that the antioxidants found in olive oil—and especially those in EVOO—can neutralize these potentially harmful free radicals. For instance, olive oil contains squalene, an oily compound that also occurs naturally in the human body. Studies show that squalene helps scavenge a type of free radical known as reactive oxygen species, or ROS. In one recent clinical trial that appeared in the journal *Bioactive Compounds in Health and Disease*, researchers found that squalene exerted significant antioxidant activity in people with type 2 diabetes. While these findings are promising, there's one problem—your body's ability to produce squalene declines with age. However, including EVOO in your diet on a regular basis may help offset this decline.

Powerful Polyphenols

Olive oil is also an incredibly abundant source of polyphenols. Polyphenols are a type of micronutrient that acts like an antioxidant, neutralizing free radicals and potentially lowering the risk of developing a number of chronic diseases. While polyphenols are largely found in fruits and vegetables, studies show that berries, chocolate, coffee, red wine, and some spices contain particularly high amounts of these protective compounds. But one of the best sources of polyphenols is extra virgin olive oil.

Although EVOO contains at least 20 different polyphenol compounds, there are five that boast an especially wide spectrum of health benefits. For instance, these specific polyphenols act like potent antioxidants that guard against free-radical damage that can cause changes to your DNA. They are also powerful anti-inflammatory compounds that reduce the systemic low-level inflammation that contributes to a range of chronic diseases. But that just scratches the surface of what these fab five polyphenols can do.

The **flavonoids** in EVOO help regulate cellular activity, and because they act like strong antioxidants, they fight off free radicals that cause oxidative stress in your body. Plus, they help reduce systemic inflammation thanks to their anti-inflammatory properties. Research also shows that one type of flavonoid called luteolin increases the body's production of collagen and helps maintain healthy bones. In one study that appeared in the *Journal of Nutritional Biochemistry*, supplementing with luteolin significantly increased bone-mineral density and bone-mineral content in the femur, which is the longest bone in the body.

Lignans, on the other hand, act like weak estrogens in the body and have been shown to lower the risk of heart disease, osteoporosis, and breast cancer. Because lignans help balance estrogen levels in the body, they've also been found to ease some of the symptoms of menopause like hot flashes and insomnia.

If you've ever wondered what gives EVOO its unique peppery bite, look no further than to another polyphenol called **oleocanthal**. Like the other polyphenolic compounds in olive oil, oleocanthal boasts potent antioxidant and anti-inflammatory benefits. But this unique polyphenol has also been found to slow the growth of cancer cells and trigger apoptosis, the natural process of programmed cell death. As a result, oleocanthal may help inhibit the spread of cancer. Other studies highlight oleocanthal's neuroprotective properties. Specifically, it reduces inflammation in the brain and helps clear beta-amyloid plaques, the proteins implicated in Alzheimer's disease. It also strengthens the blood-brain barrier against toxins. This has led some researchers to speculate that EVOO might play a role in preventing Alzheimer's and could possibly even benefit those in the early stages of the disease.

Then there's **oleuropein**, the most abundant and well-researched polyphenol in EVOO. Studies show that oleuropein has extremely strong antioxidant effects. According to Italian researchers from the University of Milan, oleuropein has antioxidant powers like vitamins C and E. But this compound, which is found only in olives and olive leaves, also reduces inflammation, decreases the risk of heart disease, helps prevent cancer, enhances cognition, protects the liver, has antidiabetic properties, and guards against harmful bacteria and viruses. Talk about a multitasking marvel!

Oleuropein's perks don't stop there. As this compound degrades, it forms another important polyphenol called **hydroxytyrosol.** Here's how it works: As olives ripen, some of the oleuropein they contain is converted to hydroxytyrosol. When you consume EVOO, the remaining oleuropein is transformed into hydroxytyrosol in your body where it works its health-promoting magic. Like oleuropein, studies show that hydroxytyrosol is a potent antioxidant and anti-inflammatory that also helps prevent cancer and cardiovascular disease, boosts brain function, enhances metabolic health, and protects against harmful bacteria that can contribute to gastrointestinal and respiratory problems. Plus, recent studies report that hydroxytyrosol helps prevent osteoporosis via its positive effect on bone formation. It's also been shown to have sight-saving benefits by contributing to the regeneration of pigment in the retina. This may, in turn, help prevent glaucoma and macular degeneration. Hydroxytyrosol may even protect the skin against damaging UV rays that can prematurely age skin.

While researchers continue to tease out all the ways this potent polyphenol can benefit health, enough is currently known to lead the European Union to recognize its health potential. As a result, European regulations dictate that an olive oil product can claim that it only provides health benefits if it contains at least 5 mg of hydroxytyrosol per 20 g (or about 2 tablespoons) of the oil.

Healthy Fats

If you think that all fats are bad, think again. EVOO consists of 80 percent monounsaturated fat, a type of fat that can reduce LDL cholesterol. Monounsaturated fatty acids (MUFA) also provide nutrients to help develop and maintain your body's cells. Plus, there is some evidence that a diet rich in MUFAs may help reduce the risk of certain cancers, especially hormone-related cancers like breast and prostate cancer.

One important type of MUFA is oleic acid, which accounts for 92 percent of the monounsaturated fat in EVOO. Classified as an omega-9 fatty acid, oleic acid is needed by the body to make sure cell membranes are thick enough to maintain proper membrane fluidity.

When it comes to specific conditions, studies show that oleic acid can decrease the risk of cardiovascular disease due to its effects on the lipids present in blood vessels. It's also been clinically found to improve blood sugar, mood, bone strength, and it may even lower the risk of cancer.

But EVOO contains both omega-3 and omega-6 fatty acids, too. These two types of fatty acids are considered essential since the body cannot produce them and they must be obtained from food or supplements. Omega-3s inhibit chronic inflammation that contributes to coronary artery disease, rheumatoid arthritis, hypertension, and even cancer. Omega-6s, on the other hand, can be either helpful or harmful depending on how much is consumed. When eaten in moderation and balanced with omega-3s, they can boost protective HDL cholesterol and lower potentially bad LDL. Omega-6s can also play an important role in brain function and promote bone, metabolic, reproductive, and skin health. The ratio of omega-6s to omega-3s typically found in a high-quality EVOO is about 8:1, which is considered moderate.

You may have heard, however, that consuming moderate to large amounts of omega-6s can be bad for your health. Yes and no. Ultra-processed foods are often made with seed oils like canola or safflower that are high in omega-6s. When these foods are processed, the oils (as well as the omega-6s they contain) become oxidized and this can spark detrimental inflammation throughout the body. But because natural sources of omega-6s, like EVOO, olives, and walnuts, aren't processed, they don't have the same pro-inflammatory effects.

Potent Phytosterols

Olive oil is also a good source of phytosterols—a group of natural compounds found in plant cell membranes. Because phytosterols are structurally similar to cholesterol, they compete with your body's cholesterol for absorption in the digestive system. As a result, cholesterol absorption can help reduce LDL cholesterol.

The primary phytosterol in olive oil is beta-sitosterol, which, along with its ability to lower cholesterol, provides antioxidant and anti-inflammatory benefits. It also supports a healthy immune response. But beta-sitosterol's benefits don't stop there. Research suggests that eating foods rich in this particular phytosterol provides antidiabetic perks by supporting better insulin sensitivity. There's also some evidence that the beta-sitosterol in olive oil may help shrink prostate size and ease symptoms in men with benign prostatic hyperplasia (an enlarged prostate).

Vitamins E and K

In addition to these healthful compounds, EVOO also contains modest amounts of vitamins E and K. Vitamin E is an essential nutrient for cardiovascular health and a robust immune system. Unlike most vitamins, however, vitamin E isn't a single nutrient. Instead, it's made up of a group of eight fat-soluble compounds. These consist of four tocopherols (alpha-, beta-, gamma-, and delta-tocopherol) and four tocotrienols (alpha-, beta-, gamma-, and delta-tocotrienol). The vitamin E in olive oil consists of tocopherols, which are powerful antioxidant and anti-inflammatory compounds shown to support healthy arteries and bones.

The vitamin K in olive oil is in the form of K1, also called phylloquinone. Studies show that K1 plays an essential role in blood clotting. What's more, according to the U.S. Department of Agriculture, this fat-soluble nutrient also has strong antioxidant and anticancer properties.

As you can see, EVOO is bursting with good nutrition. In the following chapters, we'll take a deeper dive into how the beneficial compounds and nutrients in EVOO work together to prevent or benefit various health conditions and enhance overall good health.

CHAPTER 3
The Heart-Healthy Oil

Your heart is your body's hardest-working organ, and it's the centerpiece of your cardiovascular system. Thanks to its pumping action, a healthy heart constantly circulates blood throughout the body, carrying oxygen and nutrients to your organs and tissues via a series of arteries, veins, and capillaries. When everything's working correctly, your heart is like a high-performance machine that's essential to life itself. But for many people, their heart health is less than optimal and may even be life threatening.

Despite advances in medicine, cardiovascular disease remains the leading cause of death in

America. In fact, one person dies of heart disease every 34 seconds. And these statistics don't just include older people. According to the Centers for Disease Control and Prevention (CDC), about 20 million adults between the ages of 20 and 65 have been diagnosed with some form of cardiovascular disease. Of more concern, the agency reports that about 2 in every 10 deaths from heart disease occurs in adults under the age of 65.

Are You at Risk?

While some people are genetically predisposed to develop cardiovascular disease, your age, race, and gender matter, too. Men over the age of 45 and women over the age of 55 are at an increased risk of heart disease. And the World Heart Federation notes that people with African or Asian ancestry are also at a higher risk. Although there's nothing you can do to change these risk factors, that doesn't mean you simply have to live with cardiovascular disease. Since the biggest overall risk factor for many people stems from an unhealthy lifestyle, there are plenty of things you can do to avoid becoming a statistic.

Top lifestyle threats you can change, starting today:

- A sedentary lifestyle
- An unhealthy diet filled with ultra-processed foods
- Being overweight or obese
- Chronic stress
- Depression
- Excessive alcohol consumption
- Smoking or frequent exposure to second-hand smoke
- Social isolation
- Other factors can also increase your risk, and they are often a result of these threats:
- Elevated C-reactive protein (CRP), a marker of systemic inflammation

- High LDL and/or low HDL cholesterol levels
- Hypertension
- Type 2 diabetes
- Unhealthy triglyceride levels

Fortunately, addressing the risk factors that you can change often benefits these other risk factors. Studies have conclusively shown that adopting a healthy diet and exercise routine, starting a daily meditation habit, spending time with family and friends, and quitting smoking can reduce all these downstream risk factors and conditions. But if making changes on all these fronts seems overwhelming, take heart. There's one incredibly easy change you can make that can yield big results—simply trade out all of the oils in your kitchen for a bottle of high-quality EVOO.

A growing amount of research shows that a daily dose of EVOO can help you get closer to joining the healthy-heart club by fostering better cholesterol levels, blood pressure, and weight while also reducing inflammation. In one clinical trial of 7,200 people at high risk of cardiovascular disease, researchers found that a diet supplemented with either olive oil or EVOO reduced the participant's risk by 35 percent and 39 percent respectively. The study also reported that for every 10 grams (just over a tablespoon) of EVOO the participants consumed each day, cardiovascular disease risk dropped by an impressive 10 percent.

Another large trial by the same researchers reported even better results. This trial found that, after adjusting for other factors, people who ate the most olive oil had a 19 percent lower risk of dying of cardiovascular disease compared to people who ate the least olive oil.

Your Arteries Love EVOO

Heart disease isn't a single condition. Instead, it encompasses several diseases and risk factors, including arrhythmia, atrial fibrillation, unhealthy cholesterol levels, heart failure, hypertension, and peripheral vascular disease. The unifying factor in all these conditions is something called atherosclerosis—the gradual buildup of plaques inside the arteries. Over time, this buildup can narrow and stiffen arteries. This, in turn, can slow or even block blood flow to the heart, as well as the organs and tissues throughout the body.

Think this can't happen to you? Think again! An estimated 40 percent of adults have been diagnosed with at least some plaque buildup. And another 50 percent of Americans over the age of 45 are living with this artery-compromising condition but don't know it. That's not surprising since atherosclerosis typically doesn't have any symptoms to alert you to its artery-clogging effects. Yet, even though you may not feel it, your arteries are being subjected to damaging changes every day.

Here's how it works: Atherosclerosis starts when the endothelium (the lining of blood vessels) becomes injured. This triggers the formation of plaque at the site of the damage. Plaque is a fatty substance made up of cholesterol, calcium, cellular waste, and a blood-clotting material called fibrin. Over time, these plaques accumulate, further damaging the arterial lining and causing arteries to become narrow and stiff. As they grow, plaques can eventually reduce blood flow to the heart, brain, and other parts of the body. If plaque becomes unstable it can rupture, causing a blood clot to form that can block the artery completely and trigger a heart attack or stroke.

For decades, doctors pointed to unhealthy LDL cholesterol levels as the primary cause of atherosclerosis. More current research, however, shows that the following two factors likely play an even bigger role in damaging arteries.

Inflammation is the body's natural response to injury. But when inflammation becomes chronic, it can damage the arterial walls. This is because plaque is naturally drawn to the site of inflammation. Over time, the plaque accumulation contributes to atherosclerosis. Chronic inflammation also weakens existing plaque, making it more vulnerable to bursting and causing a dangerous blockage.

Oxidation is a chemical reaction that occurs when a substance is exposed to oxygen, causing a molecule to lose one of its electrons. It's essentially the same process that causes a cut apple to turn brown. But when oxidation happens in your body, it sets off a dangerous chain reaction that can compromise the health of your arteries. More specifically, when LDL cholesterol becomes oxidized, it builds up inside your endothelium and contributes to atherosclerosis. Oxidation also triggers inflammation in the arteries, which causes even more plaque buildup.

Even though all of this may sound ominous, there is good news. EVOO can help protect against atherosclerosis in several ways. For instance, in one large cohort of three studies involving nearly 60,000 people, Spanish researchers found that those consuming EVOO had a significantly lower risk of heart attack and stroke—two potential complications of atherosclerosis. According to findings from a growing number of studies, this is because EVOO reduces the markers of inflammation (specifically CRP) and helps prevent oxidation. What's more, according to scientists at the Yale-Griffin Prevention Research Center, EVOO can actually make your arteries function better. During the randomized, controlled, double-blind, crossover study, participants were assigned to consume a daily smoothie containing 50 mL of either EVOO rich in polyphenols or a refined olive oil. By the end of the study, those drinking the EVOO smoothie experienced considerably better endothelial function than those consuming the refined olive oil, signifying less oxidation and less inflammation.

The Cholesterol Connection

Let's take a closer look at how EVOO works to improve the many aspects of cardiovascular disease, starting with cholesterol. Cholesterol, even LDL cholesterol, isn't inherently bad. In fact, your body needs cholesterol to make cell membranes, many hormones, and vitamin D.

A systematic review published in 2016 found that seniors with high LDL cholesterol levels live just as long or longer than people with low LDL. This suggests that it's not the number that matters. What does matter is the size of your LDL particles and whether they are oxidized. Small, oxidized LDL particles gravitate to any injured areas in the endothelium like flies to honey and contribute to the artery-clogging buildup of plaque. Consuming EVOO not only prevents oxidation but also increases the size of those cholesterol particles. It also boosts HDL levels—the good type of cholesterol that absorbs cholesterol in the blood and carries it back to the liver, so it can be shuttled out of the body.

Despite LDL not necessarily being the big bad boogeyman it's made out to be, some people do have cholesterol levels that are dangerously high: total cholesterol that's higher than 240 mg/dL and LDL cholesterol north of 160 mg/dL. Studies report that the monounsaturated fatty acids in EVOO can significantly reduce both total and LDL cholesterol levels. And reducing total and LDL cholesterol levels may, in turn, reduce oxidative stress and inflammation inside the arteries. As a bonus, EVOO's powerful polyphenols not only inhibit cholesterol oxidation; they also help dampen the spike in triglycerides that occurs after eating.

Help for High Blood Pressure

About half of American adults are living with high blood pressure—technically known as hypertension—and that's a problem since it's the leading cause of heart attack and stroke. Blood pressure is the amount of force (pressure) that blood exerts on the walls of the blood vessels as it passes through them. When the pressure in your blood vessels becomes too great, the walls of your arteries may narrow or thicken, worsening atherosclerosis and putting an extra burden on the heart. What's considered too high? Blood pressure that reaches 140/90 or above on a consistent basis. What do the numbers mean? The top number, or systolic pressure, represents the pressure while your heart is beating. The bottom number, or diastolic pressure, represents the pressure between beats when the heart is relaxed.

High blood pressure doesn't discriminate. It affects every social class, every race, and every age. However, certain groups are especially vulnerable to hypertension, according to the National Heart, Lung, and Blood Institute. These include men over the age of 45 and women over the age of 55, African Americans, and people with diabetes or who are overweight.

If you're looking to take the pressure off your blood vessels, EVOO can help. This was shown in a double-blind, randomized clinical trial comparing the efficacy of high polyphenol EVOO with low polyphenol EVOO. Among the 50 middle-aged people who volunteered for the trial, half consumed 60 mL of high-polyphenol EVOO each day while the other half consumed the same amount of low-polyphenol EVOO. By the end of the study, the researchers found that those taking the high-polyphenol oil experienced a 2.5 mmHg drop in their peripheral blood pressure and a 2.7 mmHg decrease in their systolic blood pressure after just three weeks.

Another trial found that high-polyphenol EVOO reduced both systolic and diastolic blood pressure in a group of young women with stage 1 hypertension. The women were assigned to consume either EVOO with 564 mg/kg of total polyphenols or a refined olive oil for eight weeks. Compared to the refined oil, the EVOO not only decreased both systolic and diastolic blood pressure; it was also more effective at combating hypertension than the DASH (Dietary Approaches to Stop Hypertension) diet.

These studies suggest that the key to bringing blood pressure into a healthier range with EVOO may lie in the oil's overall polyphenol content. But there may be one particular polyphenol compound that's especially effective for reducing both systolic and diastolic blood pressure—oleuropein. This specific polyphenol doesn't act directly on your arteries. Instead, it appears to work by protecting the hypothalamus from oxidative stress. The hypothalamus is a gland at the base of your brain that regulates a number of internal functions such as your hormones, your body temperature, and yes, your blood pressure.

So how much EVOO do you need to take to get these results? According to Mary M. Flynn, PhD, RN, LDN, associate professor of medicine at Brown University, you should consume at least two tablespoons every day to lower your blood pressure. Since a growing number of high-polyphenol EVOO products (check out the Resources section at the back of the book for a list) are hitting the market, it's easier than you might think to incorporate a full range of EVOO polyphenols into your everyday meals.

Atrial Fibrillation and Other Arrhythmias

Falling in love may make your heart skip a beat, but it's not the only thing that can affect the regularity of your heartbeat. In fact, heart palpitations—which can feel like a fluttering in the chest, a pounding or rapid heartbeat (tachycardia), a slow heartbeat (bradycardia), or even the skipping of a heartbeat—are often a sign of cardiac arrhythmia. An arrhythmia is a type of heart disorder that affects the heart's rhythm. This can be because of a problem with the heart's electrical system, a structural defect, or, most often, due to atherosclerosis.

The most common type of arrhythmia is atrial fibrillation, often known as A-fib. This form of arrhythmia refers to rapid or irregular contractions in the atria, which could lead to clots and eventually stroke or heart failure. If you've got a family history of A-fib, or you've been diagnosed with atherosclerosis, studies suggest that a daily dose of EVOO may provide some protection against developing the condition by reducing the oxidative stress that contributes to atherosclerosis. This is good news since, to date, there aren't any effective medical interventions that can directly prevent A-fib.

How effective is EVOO against an irregular heartbeat? As part of the PREDIMED trial, a group of researchers from various universities and hospitals throughout Spain assigned 6,705 people to one of three diets: a Mediterranean diet supplemented with EVOO, a Mediterranean diet supplemented with nuts, or a low-fat diet. After following the participants for nearly five years, the researchers found that EVOO was most effective for reducing the risk of developing A-fib.

EVOO may be especially beneficial for overweight individuals at risk of A-fib. In another large study involving more than 18,000 participants, researchers found that overweight participants who ate the largest amount of EVOO experienced a greater degree of protection against A-fib compared to non-overweight study subjects.

Heart Failure

If you've got congestive heart failure, your heart doesn't suddenly quit working. Instead, heart failure is a progressive condition that occurs when the heart can't efficiently pump blood throughout the body. This can cause blood and other fluids to eventually back up in your abdomen, liver, lower body, and lungs. Atherosclerosis and high blood pressure can both contribute to heart failure by boosting the odds of having a heart attack that can damage the heart muscle.

Olive oil has been found to protect the heart from damage after a heart attack, effectively slowing the progression of heart failure. Preliminary research suggests that this is due to olive oil's ability to reduce both inflammation and oxidative stress.

Peripheral Artery Disease

Peripheral artery disease (PAD), also known as peripheral vascular disease, is a painful condition that's a result of plaque buildup and reduced blood flow in the arteries in your extremities. A direct result of atherosclerosis, PAD primarily affects long-term smokers and people with type 2 diabetes. But other conditions such as high blood pressure or metabolic syndrome can also increase the risk of developing this condition.

When PAD affects the arteries in your legs, you may experience muscle pain or weakness while walking, which stops within minutes of resting. While these symptoms typically occur in more advanced cases, mild to moderate PAD might not have any warning signs. If you're at a higher risk of this form of atherosclerosis, it's wise to talk with your health-care provider—especially since untreated PAD can lead to poor wound healing, limited mobility, and even amputation.

If you do have a higher than average risk of PAD, it's also smart to consider boosting your intake of EVOO. A recent analysis of more than 4,300 people who underwent ankle-brachial index testing (a test that measures blood flow in your extremities) suggests that increasing your consumption of EVOO can help prevent PAD in those with an increased risk.

Because cardiovascular disease continues to be the No. 1 killer in America, it's important to do everything you can to reduce your risk. One of the easiest and most effective strategies you can adopt is to add EVOO to your diet. After all, research clearly shows that olive oil, and especially EVOO, really is the heart-healthy oil.

Get Heart Smart

Getting heart smart begins with understanding how this all-important organ works to keep you alive. Although your heart weighs between 8 and 14 ounces, this hollow muscle is responsible for circulating blood throughout your entire body. Your heart is divided into two halves, each designed to shuttle blood in one direction only. The right half of your heart receives the blood returning from every part of your body after the oxygen has been used by the tissues and organs. It then pumps this oxygen-deficient blood into your lungs through a vessel called the pulmonary artery. There, the blood picks up oxygen before traveling to the left half of your heart.

After this newly oxygenated blood makes its way to the left side of your heart, it is pumped into the aorta, the largest artery in your body. From there, the process starts all over again as the blood is sent to all the other arteries, veins, and capillaries in your body. During the resting period between each heartbeat, the heart also supplies blood to itself, delivering oxygen and other critical nutrients that allow it to maintain its constant pumping action.

If your heart becomes stressed, it can form alternative routes to provide blood to the undernourished heart muscle by adjusting blood flow and the signals created by the nervous system. Your heart can also grow new blood vessels. The heart's amazing adaptability, however, depends on the health of its coronary arteries, which depends on the health of each artery's inner lining.

This inner lining is made up of tissue called the endothelium. When this tissue is healthy, it maintains the normal tone of the blood vessels through its effect on the smooth muscles in the outer part of the vessel wall. The endothelium also plays an important role in controlling the stickiness of platelets (small, colorless, irregular blood cells). Although platelets help stop bleeding when you cut yourself, they can also cling to any tears in the endothelium and contribute to narrowed arteries, especially as you age. As you get older, your arteries also lose some of their elasticity and become smaller and less pliable. This causes the heart to work harder to push blood throughout the body. The result can be decreased blood flow as well as an increase in blood pressure—two factors that raise the likelihood of a heart attack or stroke. But as you'll see in this chapter, olive oil—and especially EVOO—can foster a healthier endothelium and reduce the risk factors that can threaten your cardiovascular well-being.

CHAPTER 4
EVOO's Anticancer Properties

It wasn't that long ago when being diagnosed with cancer was considered a death sentence. But thanks to modern medicine, that is no longer the case for many types of this disease, including breast, cervical, prostate, testicular, thyroid, and skin cancers—especially when caught in the early stages. And that's good news for the 23 million people who discover they've got "The Big C."

Even though science has made great strides in successfully treating many forms of cancer, going through chemotherapy or radiation is no picnic. Side effects include anemia, cognitive changes, fatigue, hair loss, a higher risk of infection, insomnia, loss of appetite, and nausea. And unless the treatment is specifically targeted, chemotherapy can damage or kill healthy cells along with the cancer cells. What's more, microscopic cancer cells can survive current treatments, opening the door for a future recurrence.

Unfortunately, too many people assume that because they are genetically predisposed or have a family history of cancer, they are destined to the same fate at some point in their lives. But while you may not be able to avoid all types of cancer—especially if you are at a higher than normal risk—there are plenty of healthy habits you can adopt to lower your risk.

Cancer Defined

Before we explore how EVOO can safely and effectively fight cancer, it's a good idea to know what you're up against. Cancer is a disease caused by an uncontrolled division of abnormal cells. When things are working as they should, your immune system seeks out and destroys any damaged cells in the body through a process known as apoptosis. This type of programmed cell death is usually quite effective. This is because your immune system acts like first responders when it detects the presence of abnormal proteins on the surface of cancer cells. Once identified, your immune system then kills the cancer cells. The problem is, this process isn't foolproof since cancer cells can sometimes block apoptosis.

Cancer cells are also incredibly sneaky. They can actually hide from the immune system. And all it takes is just one cancerous cell to sneak through the immune system's search-and-destroy mechanism. This rogue cell then becomes a prototype for other cells that share its capabilities. As these cancer cells accumulate, they can form one or more tumors. This tumor is known as the primary tumor and is named for the location where it began. For instance, a cancerous tumor that originates in breast tissue but travels to the bones (in a process called metastasis) is still called breast cancer.

But the growth and spread of cancer doesn't happen in a vacuum. Like all cells, cancer cells require "food" to grow and replicate. What's their favorite fare? Sugar, or more specifically, glucose. Because cancer cells require a lot of energy, they need a lot of glucose. A diet high in foods with a high glycemic rating—which is a system that shows how quickly foods like sweets, starchy vegetables, and ultra-refined foods affect blood sugar levels—can give cancer cells the energy they need to rapidly multiply. Although all cancers benefit from a diet high in glucose, certain types are more prone to thrive. For instance, a recent meta-analysis published in the journal *Nutrition* found a link between glucose and lung cancer. The study, which looked at nine studies involving more than 383,000 participants, reported that people who ate a diet filled with high glycemic index (GI) foods like bread, cookies, and cakes had a greater risk of lung cancer.

Of course sugar isn't the only nutrient cancer cells can use. In fact, when glucose isn't available, cancer cells can use uridine to fuel their growth. Uridine is a naturally occurring nucleic acid found in the body and in foods such as brewer's yeast, broccoli, fish, mushrooms, oats, and organ meats. While these foods are nutritious additions to a whole-foods diet in otherwise healthy people, a new study in the journal *Nature* reports that pancreatic cancer cells have the ability to switch to alternative nutrients like uridine, likely through a cancer-promoting mutation. While these findings are preliminary, many doctors caution against consuming supplemental uridine if you have been diagnosed with cancer.

Cancer cells also hijack some otherwise healthy amino acids, including arginine, glutamine, isoleucine, leucine, and valine. While all cells need these amino acids to survive, cancer cells metabolize these nutrients differently. This changes the way these nutrients impact the molecular switches that regulate DNA. It also affects the immune system's response to cancer. Instead of searching out and destroying cancer cells, these altered immune cells encourage the formation of tumors and the spread of cancer in the body. To access the glucose and nutrients that cancer cells need to thrive, tumors can also stimulate the formation of new blood vessels—a process known as angiogenesis—to feed their growth. If that weren't enough, new research suggests that tumors can co-opt existing blood vessels and use them for their malignant growth as well.

All this information may seem a bit overwhelming. But it simply goes to show just how opportunistic and devious cancer can be. Fortunately, there are a number of things you can do to outsmart cancer, even if you're at high risk. And that starts with comprehensive lifestyle changes that include a diet high in EVOO.

Potential Causes of Cancer

If you read the headlines, it might seem like everything causes cancer. The truth is, as prevalent as cancer is, its triggers aren't lurking around every corner. What should you be mindful of? Well-designed research has come up with a list of definitive factors that can increase your overall risk.

- Air pollution
- Being overweight or obese
- Exposure to radon (a naturally occurring radioactive gas)
- Heavy alcohol consumption
- Occupational exposure to cancer-causing chemicals like benzene or formaldehyde
- Smoking and exposure to second-hand smoke
- Some diseases like human papillomavirus (HPV) or hepatitis B and C
- The use of tanning beds

Preliminary studies suggest that exposure to everyday products laced with carcinogenic compounds may also increase your risk. These include cosmetics and personal-care products, common household products, and herbicides like glyphosate.

While you can't avoid all these factors, many are within your control. Changing your daily habits and opting for noncarcinogenic products is a great place to start.

The Cancer-Defying Diet

What you put in your mouth can be one of the most effective ways to sidestep cancer. According to the World Health Organization, 40 percent of all cancer cases could be prevented by eating a nutrient-rich diet.

Although no single food can prevent all cancers, study after study confirms that eating a healthy, minimally processed diet filled with high-fiber, polyphenol-rich fruits and vegetables confers a protective effect. Of particular note, cruciferous vegetables, like broccoli, cauliflower, and kale, contain a compound called sulforaphane that reduces the risk of hormone-dependent cancers like breast, colon, ovarian, and prostate. Colorful berries contain potent anthocyanins that encourage apoptosis, thus discouraging the spread of cancer cells. This can be particularly important if you're undergoing chemotherapy, since anthocyanins help reverse drug resistance in cancer cells and can increase their sensitivity to treatment.

On the flip side, eating a diet high in ultra-processed food can increase your odds of developing some form of the disease. The link is so solid that a large international study published in 2023 reports that for every 10 percentage–point increase in the amount of ultra-processed foods a person eats, there is a 2 percent increase in overall cancer risk and, more specifically, a 19 percent increase in ovarian cancer risk. Earlier investigations have found that people who eat a diet high in ultra-processed foods also have a greater risk of developing breast cancer, colorectal cancer, and gastric cancer.

As you can see, choosing your food wisely is one of the very best ways to protect against cancer. But if you're looking for foods that provide the most benefit, there's a catch. Much of what you'll find in the typical produce aisle has been heavily treated with pesticides, herbicides, and fungicides. Traces of these agricultural chemicals cling to fruits and vegetables, even when you wash your food before eating. This means you're getting minuscule doses of these cancer-causing chemicals, which make their way into your fatty (adipose) tissues. Once there, these compounds can hang out for decades, boosting your risk of cancer. Luckily, you can avoid much of this exposure by choosing certified organic food whenever possible.

The conventionally raised meat and farmed fish you eat can also harbor carcinogens. Large-scale commercially raised cattle and pigs are typically crowded in highly confined areas—a practice that increases stress and the risk of illness. In response, antibiotics and other drugs are often used as a preventive measure. While studies comparing the cancer-causing potential of conventionally raised meat versus grass-fed meat are lacking, it's suspected that—much like conventionally grown produce—that burger or pork chop you had for dinner likely harbors drug residue. Choosing grass-fed meat eliminates these contaminants. As a bonus, researchers from Duke University, the University of Utah, and the USDA report that a variety of cancer-fighting phytonutrients are considerably higher in grass-fed meat compared to conventional cuts.

There's even more evidence on the cancer-causing potential of farmed fish. Thirty years ago, researchers at Boston University and UCLA looked at the chemical contaminants found in the tanks of farm-raised fish and shellfish and speculated that eating farmed fish may indeed elevate the risk of cancer. Other studies have found high concentrations of man-made chlorinated industrial chemicals like dioxins and polychlorinated biphenyl (PCB) in farmed salmon. Although these chemicals were banned for commercial use decades ago, they can still be found in the environment—and in many of the foods that we eat every day. One of these studies suggests that routinely eating farm-raised salmon could double the risk of developing prostate cancer. The lesson here? If fish is on the menu, it's best to reduce your risk of consuming carcinogens by opting for wild-caught seafood.

Add EVOO to the Equation

If you're looking to enhance your defenses against cancer, cleaning up your diet is a great first step. But you can take it to the next level by ditching the cooking oils in your kitchen cabinet for an EVOO high in polyphenols. Indeed, consuming just 1 to 2 tablespoons of EVOO per day has been shown to reduce the risk of breast, digestive, and respiratory cancers.

In one analysis of 45 studies, Greek researchers found that people with the highest intake of EVOO had a 31 percent lower risk of developing any type of cancer. The risk of gastrointestinal cancer, in particular, was reduced by 23 percent. Studies from Greece, Italy, and Spain have also shown a 25 percent reduction in breast cancer risk. And epidemiological studies report that a diet rich in EVOO has a protective effect against endometrial, laryngeal, lung, oral, ovarian, pancreatic, and pharynx cancers.

EVOO has also been found to benefit people with chronic lymphocytic leukemia (CLL), the most common type of leukemia in adults. While 87 percent of patients survive at least five years after being diagnosed, there is no conventional medical cure. But a blind, randomized trial of patients with early-stage CLL suggests that a daily dose of EVOO effectively killed their cancer cells. During the study, the patients were divided into two groups. One group consumed 40 mL (a little less than 3 tablespoons) of EVOO high in polyphenols for three months while the other group consumed the same amount of EVOO low in polyphenols. After a washout period, all the participants were given 40 mL of the high-polyphenol EVOO for six months. By the end of the study, the researchers found that consuming a high-polyphenol EVOO induced apoptosis of CLL cancer cells. While more research needs to be done, these are very promising findings for anyone suffering from this type of leukemia.

What makes EVOO so effective against cancer? In a word, oleocanthal—that powerful phenolic compound found only in EVOO. Laboratory and human studies have determined that oleocanthal selectively kills cancer cells while leaving healthy cells alone. Few other cancer treatments can make this claim. These studies also show that the amount of oleocanthal in the oil matters. In other words, the more oleocanthal in EVOO, the more killing power it has.

But how exactly does oleocanthal eradicate cancer cells so effectively? In a 2019 study, researchers at Hunter College in New York City discovered that oleocanthal damages a cancer cell's lysosomes (organelles that digests old or unwanted parts of a cell, turning them into waste) by essentially poking holes in them. This causes the cellular waste to leak into the cancer cell, killing it. The process is so effective that after applying oleocanthal to the cancer cells, the Hunter researchers found that the cancer cells died within an hour—considerably faster than the body's own system of programmed cell death.

But best of all, oleocanthal doesn't harm healthy cells. This is because, unlike in healthy cells, the lysosomes in cancer cells are big, which means they contain a lot more waste. They are also quite fragile compared to the lysosomes in healthy cells, so it's easy for oleocanthal to make quick work of cancer cells—and all without triggering the side effects common to traditional chemotherapy. While these findings are preliminary, this vulnerability has some experts looking at oleocanthal-rich EVOO as a safe and effective way to fight cancer. At the very least, it's a great tool to add to other preventive measures if you have a family history of cancer or are at a higher risk for developing the disease in the future.

CHAPTER 5
EVOO's Brain Benefits

If you ask people over the age of 50 what health problem worries them most, you might be surprised at their answer. It's not cancer or heart disease. It's Alzheimer's. And their fears might not be unfounded. Currently, more than six million Americans are living with this brain-robbing disease. That translates to about one in every nine people over the age of 65. The Alzheimer's Association projects that number could reach 12.7 million by the year 2050.

The most frightening thing about Alzheimer's is that there is no cure. That's not to say scientists haven't tried to find answers. But so far, pharmaceutical interventions have only succeeded in temporarily slowing Alzheimer's and other forms of dementia while bringing on a host of side effects. This has left aging Americans with few answers. Instead, every time they misplace their keys or can't recall a familiar name, they worry that it could be an early sign of cognitive decline. But where drugs have failed, a growing number of studies show that EVOO has remarkable success in preventing, improving, and even reversing the cognitive decline seen in Alzheimer's and dementia.

"As ridiculous as it sounds, that means that olive oil alone has a better track record of protecting brain health than most of our approved Alzheimer's drugs," notes Dale Bredesen, MD, an internationally recognized expert in the mechanisms of neurodegenerative diseases and author of The End of Alzheimer's. This is probable because, unlike pharmaceuticals that focus only on one element of Alzheimer's and other types of neurodegeneration, EVOO successfully targets multiple brain functions and structures to preserve cognition and memory. And it does so without any of the side effects that commonly occur with the current array of Alzheimer's drugs.

Mind Matters

Before we look at the many ways EVOO can benefit the brain, let's get acquainted with this fascinating organ. Your brain orchestrates your every movement, reflex, and thought every minute of every day. It controls your body temperature, blood pressure, heart rate, and breathing. As the command center of the entire nervous system, your brain also directs your muscles and nerves, and processes a never-ending flood of information about the world around you. It sorts and stores memories, allows you to make decisions, and gives you the ability to communicate through speech. This remarkable organ also makes it possible to dream and experience emotions. All these tasks are coordinated, controlled, and regulated by an organ that weighs just three pounds.

The brain can be divided into three areas: the forebrain, the cerebellum, and the brain stem. Each area is associated with a distinct set of functions.

Your **forebrain** houses the cerebrum, which contains the cerebral cortex—an area that is responsible for all higher functions like reasoning and problem solving.

The cerebral cortex itself contains four regions that perform different tasks:

- The **frontal lobe** sits right behind your forehead, at the front of the cerebral cortex and is responsible for performing executive functions such as problem-solving. Your frontal lobe contains a region that plans and executes movement, and it's also responsible for speech, language processing, and language comprehension.
- The **parietal lobe** sits at the top of your head, right behind the frontal lobe. This is the area of the brain that interprets sensations like touch or pain that occur anywhere on or in your body. Your parietal lobe plays a key role in how you understand where things are around you (spatial orientation), as well as speech, language development, and attention.

- The **temporal lobe** is situated below the frontal and parietal lobes (toward the ears), and above the hindbrain (the bottom area of the brain at the back of the head). The temporal lobe is where the majority of sensory processing occurs, especially hearing and vision. The temporal lobe also contains the hippocampus, which plays a key role in the formation of long-term memories.
- The **occipital lobe** sits at the back of the skull and above the hindbrain. This region contains the primary visual cortex and is critical for sight.

The forebrain is also where you'll find the thalamus and the hypothalamus. The thalamus acts like a switchboard for the brain. Most sensory information passes through this area before traveling to the cerebral cortex. The hypothalamus secretes hormones that regulate your neurological and endocrine systems. It also controls basic survival responses, such as the fight-or-flight response, hunger, and thirst.

The **cerebellum** is the main structure of the hindbrain, situated at the base of the brain and at the top of the spinal cord. The cerebellum controls balance and physical stability. It is involved in motor coordination and the development of "muscle memory."

The **brain stem** is the most primitive part of the brain and includes three areas: the midbrain, the pons, and the medulla oblongata. The midbrain is involved in processing information that governs sight and sound. It also controls eye movement. The pons helps coordinate breathing, blood pressure, sleep, and waking. The medulla oblongata connects the brain to the spinal cord and controls the most basic bodily functions, such as breathing and blood circulation.

While all regions of the brain are critical for proper brain function, your neurons (nerve cells) are really running the show—and this is where things get a little complicated. Here's why: The human brain consists of approximately 100 billion neurons, which are basically on/off switches. If a neuron is turned on, it shoots an electrical signal through a wire-like axon. When the signal gets to the end of the axon, it stimulates tiny sacs that release chemicals known as neurotransmitters. These neurotransmitters then cross a gap called a synapse and attach themselves to receptors on the neighboring cell. At any given moment, millions of these neurons are sending messages via synapses to various parts of your body, causing a multitude of voluntary and involuntary reactions. The problem is, in those with Alzheimer's and other forms of dementia, this neuronal communication is disrupted. As a result, there is a reduction in key neurotransmitters, and this leads to the death of neurons.

Currently, researchers have identified about 50 neurotransmitters—and each of them is responsible for multiple tasks. But only a handful play a role in dementia and other neurological diseases.

1. **Acetylcholine:** This neurotransmitter stimulates muscles, including the muscles in your gastrointestinal tract. Acetylcholine is also important for learning and memory, and it plays a role in scheduling REM sleep. People with Alzheimer's disease have been found to have a 70–80 percent loss of this critical neurotransmitter.
2. **Dopamine:** Dopamine controls the brain's reward and pleasure centers and helps regulate movement and emotional responses. There's some evidence that Alzheimer's patients experience a reduction in dopamine, which may contribute to the behavioral problems they develop. The loss of dopamine in certain parts of the brain also causes the muscle rigidity that occurs in Parkinson's patients.
3. **Endorphin:** Known as the body's "feel good" brain chemical, endorphins are involved with pleasure. They also regulate pain and stress, modulate appetite, trigger the release of sex hormones, and enhance immunity. But multiple studies have found that people with Alzheimer's have low levels.
4. **Gamma-aminobutyric acid (GABA):** As the primary inhibitory neurotransmitter in the brain, GABA plays a significant role in brain aging and neurodegenerative disorders, including Alzheimer's disease. People who

often feel apprehensive may have low levels of GABA—and that includes people with dementia.

5. **Glutamate:** This is the most common neurotransmitter in the brain, and it's involved in most aspects of cognition, memory, and learning. It's also important for cellular metabolism, and it can provide energy to the brain. The problem is, too much glutamate in the brain can cause nerve cells to become overexcited, and this can damage or even destroy brain cells. Not surprisingly, Alzheimer's patients have an excess of glutamate in their brains.
6. **Norepinephrine:** Important for attentiveness, emotions, sleep, dreaming, and learning, norepinephrine production is often glitchy in people with dementia. This leads to low levels that contribute to the cognitive and behavioral changes that occur during the course of the disease. Both high and low levels of this neurotransmitter also play a role in mood disorders such as bipolar disorder.
7. **Serotonin:** This brain chemical acts as a catalyst for a number of functions like learning and memory. It also regulates body temperature, mood, emotion, sleep, and appetite. Too little serotonin, which is often seen in dementia patients, can lead to

depression, problems with anger control, and obsessive-compulsive disorder.

The Aging Brain

As we get older, the speed at which we process information, as well as our working and long-term memory, naturally declines. Add the fact that the parts of the brain dedicated to these functions actually shrink in size, and it is no wonder we worry about cognitive decline with each passing birthday. But things may not be quite as dire as they seem.

Until recently, brain aging was thought to occur because neurons died or stopped functioning. Neuroscientists believed that you were born with a certain number of neurons, and as you got older, some of these neurons were lost. But new research shows that dopamine controls the formation of new neurons deep in the center of the adult brain. Once born, they move to areas of the brain associated with higher brain function. Yet, even though you form new neurons throughout life, it doesn't mean that your brain won't change as you age. Over the years, brain weight and volume decrease. In fact, between age 20 and age 90, the brain loses 5 to 10 percent of its weight. Bad habits like smoking and not being active, as well as diseases like type 2 diabetes, can accelerate this shrinkage.

Diet matters too. A nutrient-poor diet filled with sugar, refined grains, and unhealthy fats (think the

Standard American Diet) contributes to atherosclerosis, which can reduce blood flow to the brain. This causes the brain to utilize oxygen and protein less efficiently. How harmful can a steady diet of ultra-processed food be? In one 2022 study of 10,775 individuals, Brazilian researchers found that men and women who ate the most ultra-processed foods had a 28 percent faster rate of global cognitive decline and a 25 percent faster rate of executive function decline compared with the participants who ate the least.

These factors can pave the way for mild cognitive impairment (MCI), which is a precursor to Alzheimer's disease. Think of it as a transitional state between the cognitive changes of normal aging and very early dementia.

According to the Mayo Clinic, symptoms of MCI may include problems with memory, language, or judgment. And this condition is not that uncommon. Studies show that MCI affects up to 19 percent of people over the age of 65. But even if you've been diagnosed with this condition, it may not inevitably lead to Alzheimer's or other dementias.

If MCI does transition to some form of dementia, a person will experience progressive changes in the brain that lead to the unhealthy accumulation of beta-amyloid and tau proteins. Alzheimer's and other types of dementia also cause the brain to shrink and brain cells to die. What's more, people with Alzheimer's disease have also been shown to have a compromised blood-brain barrier—a condition known as "leaky brain" syndrome. Together, these neurological changes result in the gradual decline in memory, thinking, behavioral, and social skills. Eventually, a dementia patient loses the ability to function and requires round-the-clock care.

10 SIGNS OF DEMENTIA

Those senior moments are typically nothing to worry about. But if you find that memory problems are interfering with daily life, it's wise to see a doctor. Catching cognitive changes in the early stages allows you to make healthy lifestyle adjustments that can potentially boost brain function.

According to the Alzheimer's Association, the most common signs of MCI, early-stage Alzheimer's disease, and other types of dementia include:

- Forgetting important dates or events; asking the same question over and over
- Being disoriented about the day, time, or place
- Difficulty following recipes or paying monthly bills
- Experiencing sudden mood swings; experiencing fear or agitation
- Having problems with vision that interfere with balance or reading
- Inability to remember familiar words when speaking or writing

- Losing interest in social activities
- Misplacing things and losing the ability to retrace one's steps
- Neglecting personal hygiene; using poor judgment regarding money
- Problems completing familiar tasks such as grocery shopping

Have You Heard?

If you have hearing loss, you have a greater chance of developing dementia, according to a 2020 Lancet commission report that lists hearing loss as one of the top risk factors for all types of dementia. The study found that compared to participants without hearing loss, people with untreated hearing loss had a 29 percent increased risk for dementia. However, no increased risk was seen in people who used hearing aids. The takeaway? If you find yourself turning up the volume on the TV, or if you frequently have to ask people to repeat themselves, don't pass it off as simple aging. Get checked out by a qualified audiologist.

EVOO for Better Brain Health

In addition to improving your overall diet, exercising regularly, and treating any underlying health conditions, adding a daily dose of EVOO is perhaps the very best thing you can do to protect your brain and lower the risk of cognitive decline as you age. This is because EVOO is able to address a number of factors that contribute to cognitive decline. Pharmaceuticals, on the other hand, focus only on temporarily improving symptoms by preventing the breakdown of acetylcholine or by reducing amyloid plaque in the brain. Amyloid plaques have become the holy grail in Alzheimer's research, yet a growing number of independent researchers note that this singular focus may be missing the bigger picture since emerging science increasingly suggests that dementia is likely the result of a variety of factors, not just one.

What's more, beta-amyloid itself may not be the problem it's made out to be. As researchers from Ohio State University point out, the beta-amyloid protein is actually beneficial, protecting the body from infections, repairing leaks in the blood-brain barrier, promoting recovery from injury, and regulating synaptic function. Problems arise when there's an overproduction of these proteins. When beta-amyloid levels are too high, the brain may not be able to clear them efficiently. And because these proteins are chemically "sticky," they can clump together and form the plaques seen in the brains of Alzheimer's patients. Even small clumps might block communication between nerve cells. Adding insult to injury, amyloid plaques could also activate the immune system, triggering an inflammatory response that devours some neurons.

Over the past 20 years, researchers have latched on to the hypothesis that ridding the brain of excess beta-amyloid would cure Alzheimer's disease. But increasingly, it looks like other changes may be at play. This could be why the current Alzheimer's drugs are so ineffective. But study after study confirms that where these drugs fail, EVOO effectively protects the brain from cognitive decline and dementia. These findings could explain why the Mediterranean diet, which is high in polyphenol-rich EVOO, has been shown to reduce the risk of dementia. It's so effective that according to a recent study that appeared in the online journal *eLife*, people who adhere to this way of eating for at least 18 months have brains that are 9 months younger than people who eat a standard "healthy" diet.

An earlier study, which was published in the *Journal of the American College of Cardiology*, got even more specific in its findings. According to the study's researchers, consuming EVOO protects memory and learning ability while also reducing the formation of beta-amyloid plaques and neurofibrillary (tau) tangles in the brain. The oil was so effective that the study's participants who consumed the most EVOO had a 29 percent lower risk of dying of Alzheimer's or other neurodegenerative diseases. Previous animal research found that EVOO enhanced working and spatial memory, as well as learning skills—benefits that also applied to this human study.

What is it about EVOO that triggers these improvements? The researchers concluded that the benefits were due to the oil's ability to reduce brain inflammation and activate autophagy, a process in which a cell breaks down and destroys old, damaged, or abnormal proteins, and recycles the useful cellular components that remain.

But quelling inflammation and boosting autophagy are just two of the ways EVOO benefits the brain. As mentioned earlier, EVOO enhances the blood-brain barrier (BBB). The blood-brain barrier is an intricate network of blood vessels and tissue made up of closely spaced cells designed to prevent harmful substances from reaching the brain while allowing water, oxygen, carbon dioxide, and general anesthetics in. It's a great system—when it works. But this protective barrier begins to break down in people with MCI or early Alzheimer's disease, allowing bacteria, toxins, and other damaging compounds to enter the brain.

Fortunately, a small randomized, controlled study of people diagnosed with MCI found that EVOO improves BBB permeability. Half the participants were given about 3 tablespoons of EVOO every day for six months while the other half consumed the same amount of refined olive oil. At the end of the study, those in the EVOO group not only had improved BBB permeability; the researchers found that EVOO resulted in better connectivity between neurons and enhanced clearance of beta-amyloid in the brain. This also led to better dementia and behavioral scores among those taking the EVOO. Although participants in the refined olive oil group saw some improvement in their cognitive scores, they didn't receive the BBB benefits or any clearance of beta-amyloids.

Because EVOO is so rich in antioxidants, it also reduces oxidative stress that may trigger changes in the brain that contribute to dementia. Oxidative stress creates free radicals, which you'll recall are molecules with an unbalanced number of electrons that can damage cells. Several studies have found that people with Alzheimer's disease have lesions in the brain caused by free-radical damage. Having a dietary protector like EVOO in your anti-Alzheimer's arsenal can help address yet another risk factor for dementia. It's so effective that research in the *Journal of Food Science and Technology* found that EVOO even protects the brain from oxidative damage caused by exposure to 2,4-dichlorophenoxyacetic acid, an herbicide found in many highly toxic weed killers.

Moreover, the phenols in EVOO—especially oleocanthal—appear to improve brain plasticity in people with MCI. What's brain plasticity? Essentially, it's an umbrella term used to describe the brain's ability to change, reorganize, and grow neural networks in response to things like new information or an injury. Brain plasticity is impaired in people with dementia. However, researchers at the Alzheimer's Center at Temple University Lewis Katz School of Medicine found that EVOO significantly improves brain plasticity and synaptic activity. And that can improve memory. The Temple scientists also confirmed that EVOO reduces inflammation in the brain.

But what really got these researchers excited was the discovery that EVOO activates autophagy. Because autophagy breaks down and clears out cellular debris, it can reduce amyloid plaques and tau tangles—at least in animals. As a result, memory and synaptic activity might be preserved. While much more research needs to be done to verify that this also occurs in humans, these preliminary findings are significant since some experts suspect that a reduction in autophagy might mark the beginning of Alzheimer's disease.

What is clear is that there's a lot more to Alzheimer's than just the accumulation of amyloid plaques. By continuing to focus solely on this one disease marker, conventional treatment may never meet expectations. But because EVOO works on so many fronts—from reducing oxidative stress and inflammation to improving autophagy, BBB permeability, and brain plasticity—it's not surprising that extra virgin olive oil is proving to be more effective than current pharmaceuticals in the fight against dementia.

CHAPTER 6
The Diabetes-Defying Power of EVOO

Type 2 diabetes. It's a condition in which the body's ability to use carbohydrates for energy is impaired by inefficient insulin function. It's also the fastest-growing disease in America. And that's a problem since type 2 diabetes can shorten your life by as much as a decade. This is because type 2 diabetes greatly increases the risk of developing atherosclerosis, cancer, coronary heart disease, erectile dysfunction, kidney disease, nerve disorders, peripheral artery disease, stroke, and vision loss.

According to the CDC, more than 37 million people living in the U.S. have type 2 diabetes. Of those, an estimated 8.5 million haven't been diagnosed or treated. Another 96 million suffer from prediabetes, a condition in which blood glucose levels are higher than normal but not high enough to be classified as full-blown diabetes. What's behind this looming diabetes epidemic? The spiraling rate of obesity in America plays a significant role. But even if you're not overweight, eating a diet high in processed foods, guzzling gallons of sugary drinks, and living a sedentary lifestyle can set you up for type 2 diabetes, especially as you age. Let's take a closer look at this insidious yet preventable disease.

Diabetes Can Be Deadly

Patients with type 2 diabetes have triple the risk of a heart attack and are 20 times more likely to have a leg amputated.

Did You Know?

Type 2 diabetes is often simply referred to as diabetes. But even though it accounts for 90-95 percent of all cases of diabetes, it's not the only type of diabetes. There is also type 1. Here's how they differ: In type 2 diabetes, an adequate amount of blood sugar–lowering insulin is produced, but the body can't use it efficiently. In type 1 diabetes (also known as insulin-dependent diabetes), a malfunction of the immune system leads to destruction of the insulin-producing cells in the pancreas, so little or no insulin is produced.

Deconstructing Type 2 Diabetes

Type 2 diabetes is a long-term condition in which the body doesn't use insulin properly to deliver glucose (blood sugar) to cells. Insulin is a hormone made in the pancreas. Its role is to lower glucose levels in the bloodstream and to promote the storage of glucose in fat, muscle, and liver cells so it can be used for energy. But if you become resistant to insulin, your muscle, fat, and liver cells can't properly respond to the hormone. As a result, these cells can't easily absorb glucose from the bloodstream. This creates a demand for higher and higher amounts of insulin to shove glucose into the resistant cells. The pancreas tries to keep up with the body's increased demand by producing more and more insulin. Eventually, however, the pancreas can't keep up, and excess glucose builds up in the bloodstream. Many people with insulin resistance have high levels of both blood glucose and insulin circulating in their blood at the same time.

What causes insulin resistance? The main factors include a diet high in ultra-processed foods, excess body fat—especially around your midsection, and a lack of physical activity. When these factors form the core of your everyday habits, your risk of developing type 2 diabetes skyrockets. And of these, being overweight or obese is the biggest driver of the disease.

Of course, obesity is just one of the risk factors for type 2 diabetes. Others include:

- Family history. The risk of type 2 diabetes increases if a parent or sibling has the disease.
- Race. Although it's unclear why, Blacks, Latinos, Native Americans, and Asian Americans are more likely to develop type 2 diabetes.
- Age. The risk increases as you get older, especially after age 45.
- Gestational diabetes. If you develop gestational diabetes when pregnant or if you give birth to a baby weighing more than 9 pounds, you are at increased risk.
- Polycystic ovary syndrome. This common condition, which is characterized by irregular menstrual periods, excessive hair growth, and obesity, also increases the risk of diabetes.

Diagnosing Diabetes

Full-blown type 2 diabetes has some distinct symptoms including blurred vision, fatigue, frequent thirst, itchiness in the genital area, unexplained weight loss, urinating more often than normal, and slow wound healing. But the symptoms of prediabetes and early-stage type 2 diabetes are often absent or can simply fly under the radar. At this stage of the game, the only way to know if you're on the path toward diabetes is with testing. Diagnostic testing may include:

- **Hemoglobin A1C test.** This test, which is also called a glycosylated hemoglobin test, measures your average blood glucose levels for the previous three months. A normal HbA1c level is below 5.7 percent. A level between 5.7 and 6.4 percent signals prediabetes. And a level of 6.5 percent or more indicates diabetes.
- **Fasting plasma glucose test.** This test measures how much glucose is in your plasma. You will need to fast for eight hours before taking it. A fasting blood sugar level of 99 mg/dL or lower is normal. A range of 100-125 mg/dL points to prediabetes. And 126 mg/dL or higher indicates that you have diabetes.
- **Oral glucose tolerance test.** During this test, your blood is drawn three times: before, one hour after, and two hours after you drink a dose of glucose. The test results show how well your body deals with glucose before and after the drink. A plasma glucose level under 140 mg/dL after two hours is considered normal. The two-hour plasma glucose level of 140-199 mg/dL implies impaired glucose tolerance. The two-hour plasma glucose level of 200 mg/dL or higher indicates diabetes.

Once you have your results, you can work with your health-care provider on a treatment strategy. While a variety of medications can help manage your blood sugar levels and improve your insulin sensitivity, they often carry a range of side effects. Depending on the severity of your condition, you may want to consider a lifestyle approach first. According to a National Institutes of Health survey, simple lifestyle changes such as diet and exercise can reduce the risk of diabetes by 58 percent. They can also improve—and may even eliminate—existing type 2 diabetes.

Improve Insulin Sensitivity and Glucose Uptake with EVOO

When it comes to diabetes, one of the easiest ways to prevent becoming one of the statistics is by adding EVOO to your everyday routine. If you're living with type 2 diabetes, EVOO can also help you manage your disease. This was shown in a 2017 assessment of 4 studies and 29 clinical trials published in the journal Nutrition & Diabetes. The review noted that people with the highest consumption of EVOO had the most significant drop in HbA1c and fasting plasma glucose, resulting in a 16 percent lower risk of developing type 2 diabetes. A more recent review involving over 800,000 individuals found even better results. In this study, those with the highest EVOO intake had a 22 percent lower risk.

What these reviews discovered was that eating meals containing EVOO lowered glucose levels in the blood and triggered a greater release of insulin compared to meals without the oil. These two actions ensure that cells can effectively utilize blood glucose without overwhelming the pancreas. EVOO also lowered triglycerides and promoted the intestinal absorption of dietary fat.

The secret to EVOO's beneficial impact on diabetes lies in the polyphenols the oil contains, especially hydroxytyrosol and oleuropein. Preclinical research reports that these two antioxidants not only prevent oxidative damage but also improve glucose transport, thus reducing glucose in the bloodstream. They also promote the release of insulin by the pancreas, enhance insulin sensitivity, and decrease the absorption of carbohydrates.

More Ways to Prevent and Reverse Diabetes Naturally

In addition to EVOO, adopting a healthy diet is key. This is because, at its core, type 2 diabetes is a nutritional disease. As such, the foods you eat can play a critical role in either fostering or preventing the disease. Diets high in ultra-processed foods, drinks with added sugars, and even fruit juice promote elevated fasting blood sugar and lead to insulin resistance, weight gain, and an increased risk of diabetes. Opting instead for foods that help keep your blood sugar on an even keel can reduce your risk. Among the best are those low on the glycemic index.

Tame Your Sugar Dragon

If you've ever tried (and failed) to cut back on sugar, don't think it's due to a lack of willpower. According to researchers at Princeton University, sugar hijacks your brain, affecting your natural reward centers and making it just as addictive as cocaine or heroin. But getting your sugar fix doesn't just affect your brain. Sugar also sends your blood sugar levels on a wild roller coaster ride, setting you up for insulin resistance and type 2 diabetes. In fact, drinking just one or two sugary drinks each day can increase your risk by 26 percent. Here are some easy ways to loosen sugar's hold over your health:

- **Reduce the amount of sugar you eat gradually**. Going "cold turkey" can trigger cravings. If you normally take 2 teaspoons of sugar in your coffee, cut down to one and a half teaspoons for a week, then one, then one half. Eventually, you'll get to the point when you don't need sugar at all.
- **Know all the names for sugar**. Common names for sugar include brown sugar, corn

syrup, dextrin, dextrose, fructose, fruit juice concentrate, high-fructose corn syrup, galactose, glucose, honey, hydrogenated starch, invert sugar maltose, lactose, mannitol, maple syrup, molasses, polyols, raw sugar, sorghum, sucrose, sorbitol, and turbinado.

- **Watch out for hidden sugar**. Cough syrups, chewing gum, tomato sauce, baked beans, soups, salad dressings, and lunch meats often contain hidden sugar. Check ingredient labels for added sugar that may be lurking in your food.

Filling your plate with minimally processed nutrient-rich foods that rank low on the GI scale is the best way to prevent diabetes. It's also the best way to manage your blood sugar if you've already been diagnosed with either prediabetes or diabetes. Antioxidant-rich vegetables should be the mainstay of every meal since they provide a wealth of beneficial fiber, vitamins, minerals, and other healthy phytochemicals. Plus, because most nonstarchy vegetables have a low GI, you can take an "all you can eat" approach.

Adding 4 to 6 ounces of high-quality protein like grass-fed beef, organic free-range chicken, wild-caught fish, or pastured eggs to each meal helps keep your blood sugar stable and your appetite satisfied. One clinical trial in the journal *Diabetes* found that patients who ate a high-protein, low-carbohydrate diet experienced a dramatic drop in the amount of glucose circulating through their bloodstream. This led the researchers to conclude that this way of eating may help some patients manage their blood sugar issues without the need for drugs.

According to a more recent study that appeared in *Frontiers in Nutrition*, eating a high-protein diet lowers your postprandial glucose response—how your body responds to sugar and starch after you eat a meal. It does this by enhancing the release of insulin and improving the body's ability to use that insulin.

How much protein do you need? Although current recommendations advise consuming 0.8 grams per kilogram of weight each day (g/kg/day), that amount was set using outdated studies of healthy young men. If you're not in that group—and especially if you're an older adult—it's likely that amount of dietary protein isn't enough. Instead, recent studies recommend eating upwards of 1.0 to 1.5 g/kg/day. For someone weighing 150 pounds, that translates to a daily intake of 68 to 102 grams of protein per day.

Boosting your protein also slows age-related muscle breakdown, accelerates fat oxidation, and improves body composition. And these benefits are amplified when protein is combined with a regular exercise program. Indeed, if there were anything close to a magic bullet for preventing or reversing type 2 diabetes, exercise is it. Exercise improves the uptake of glucose by your skeletal muscle while enhancing both insulin sensitivity and the disposal of excess glucose. It's also been shown to increase the density of insulin receptors and lower HbA1c levels. Plus, it reduces the risk of diabetic complications like peripheral artery disease and heart attack.

For the most benefit from exercise, intensity matters. This was shown in one analysis of nine randomized trials conducted at the University of Ottawa. During their analysis, the researchers found that people with type 2 diabetes who participated in 20 weeks of moderate exercise experienced a marked improvement in their HbA1c levels. But the researchers also reported that people who participated in intense exercise such as high-intensity interval training (HIIT) had even better blood glucose control than those who exercised moderately.

What type of exercise is best? While aerobic exercise has long been recommended for people with diabetes, new research clearly shows that resistance training is even more effective for improving glycemic control. In one review of 14 trials involving 668 people at risk of type 2 diabetes, participating in resistance training (using free weights, weight machines, or resistance bands) two to four times per week led to significant reductions in HbA1c and fasting plasma glucose, as well as better body fat percentages and cholesterol levels.

Similar results were found in an even larger meta-analysis involving 1,172 patients who had been diagnosed with type 2 diabetes. In this study, however, the researchers also made a direct link between improved muscle strength and reduced HbA1c levels.

If you're new to exercise, check with your health-care provider before you begin. This is especially important if you're already living with diabetes. The UCLA David Geffen School of Medicine recommends checking your blood glucose levels 15 to 30 minutes before your workout, and again every 30 to 60 minutes during exercise. If your levels are higher than 250 mg/dL, check for ketone. If present, do not exercise. On the other hand, if your levels are less than 100 mg/dL, eat a snack before your workout. It's also smart to carry a fast-acting carbohydrate-rich snack with you to treat an unexpected drop in your blood sugar.

Drink Up!

Make sure to drink plenty of water while exercising because dehydration can adversely affect blood sugar levels.

Whether you're attempting to avoid becoming insulin resistant or actively trying to manage type 2 diabetes, look to lifestyle fixes first. Pairing EVOO with a nutrient-rich high-protein diet and regular workouts that prioritize resistance training can effectively keep diabetes at bay in those at high risk and improve the condition in those who have been diagnosed with the disease.

CHAPTER 7
EVOO for Better Joint Health

We often take our joints for granted until we wake up one morning with a little stiffness when getting out of bed. While it might be easy to ignore at first, at some point that stiffness can turn to pain that makes everyday activities like taking a walk or climbing the stairs into a challenge. Welcome to arthritis.

Osteoarthritis (OA) is one of the most common chronic health problems in America today, affecting more than 58 million people. That's one in every four adults. And as an increasing number of baby boomers and Gen Xers head into their senior years, those numbers are anticipated to keep going up. In fact, the Centers for Disease Control and Prevention estimates that number will hit 78 million by the year 2040.

Aging and Your Joints

Why are your joints so vulnerable to problems as you age? To understand the connection between age and arthritis, you should become familiar with how your joints work when they're healthy.

Your joints are the places where your bones come together to allow for coordinated movement. There are 206 bones in the human skeleton, and the vast majority of them come together in joints, where a cavity filled with a thick, slimy fluid called synovial fluid separates the bones from each other. Cartilage—spongy tissue on the end of each bone—covers the bone surfaces where they connect, allowing them to effortlessly glide one bone over the other. This cartilage is made of two types of molecules: proteoglycans and collagen. Proteoglycans provide elasticity and resiliency to your joints, whereas collagen provides strength.

But, as you age, your body's production of both of these proteins' declines. As a result, cartilage begins to break down. Your immune system sees this deterioration as an injury and sends out pro-inflammatory compounds called prostaglandins to fix the problem. But since the body can't produce enough proteoglycans and collagen to support your joints, cartilage continues to break down. This causes the immune system to send out a steady flow of prostaglandins. But now, instead of healing this ongoing injury, these prostaglandins create excessive inflammation that can further damage joints.

Making matters worse, this deterioration of cartilage causes more pressure on the bones. The joint then responds by producing excessive amounts of synovial fluid. This excess can then lead to swelling of the joint cavity. And this can trigger pain and joint stiffness. Adding insult to injury, as cartilage wears away, the bone underneath also responds by thickening. This produces irregularities and causes the surface of the bone to become rough or bumpy, contributing to even more pain and inflammation, especially during joint movement.

Osteoarthritis: Are You at Risk?

There are more than 100 different types of arthritis, with OA being the most prevalent. Over time, people with OA can experience so much cartilage loss that bone begins to rub against bone, causing severe disability—especially if it goes untreated.

Even if your OA doesn't get to that point, the condition can cause significant joint pain and stiffness, a loss of flexibility, reduced range of motion, visible inflammation, bone spurs, and a grating, crackling, or popping sound when you move the affected joint. And while OA can impact any of the 360 joints in your body, the most commonly affected areas include your hands, fingers, shoulders, neck, lower back, hips, and knees.

Age is the biggest risk factor for joint deterioration. This is because the longer you live, the more repetitive stress your joints will endure. People who have experienced a past injury such as torn cartilage or a dislocated joint also have a higher risk of developing OA. This is common among both professional and amateur athletes.

People who are obese or who have poor posture are also at an increased risk.

But there are other risk factors that can affect anyone. These include having a family member with the condition, particularly parents or sibling; being a woman, especially after menopause; or having an occupation that involves kneeling, climbing, heavy lifting, or similar actions.

Diagnosing and Treating OA

Although it can be easy to ignore a little joint pain or stiffness, it's important to see a doctor for a proper diagnosis. This is because OA can lead to other health complications, such as poor sleep, weight gain because of limited mobility, erosion of your ligaments and tendons, hairline fractures, bleeding in the area around the joint, and even bone death.

Along with a general exam, your health-care provider will likely check your reflexes and look at the problem joint. X-rays are often ordered because they can show a loss of joint space, bone damage, bone remodeling, or bone spurs. In some cases, an MRI (magnetic resonance imaging) will also be ordered. MRIs can show any damage to the soft tissues in and around the joint. Finally, your health-care provider may want blood tests to rule out other causes for your symptoms.

There is no cure for OA, but it can be managed. If you are diagnosed with the condition, treatment typically depends on the severity of your symptoms. Exercise or physical therapy may be recommended to improve pain and joint function. If you are overweight or obese, you may also be advised to lose weight. This helps take the pressure off joints—especially in your knees, hips, and lower back.

Conventional treatment also includes drugs like pain relievers, steroids, or even antidepressants. Pain relievers fall into two categories: over-the-counter (OTC) pain relievers and prescription nonsteroidal anti-inflammatory drugs (NSAIDs). OTC medications include acetaminophen (e.g., Tylenol) or NSAIDs like ibuprofen or naproxen (e.g., Advil or Aleve, respectively). While these drugs can offer temporary relief, they come with some long-lasting and potentially serious side effects. For example, acetaminophen can cause symptoms of an allergic reaction, including rash, hives, itching, hoarseness, difficulty breathing or swallowing, and swelling of the face, throat, tongue, lips, eyes, hands, feet, ankles, or lower legs. NSAIDs, on the other hand, can cause gastrointestinal upset, headache, dizziness, and drowsiness. Long-term use can also contribute to ulcers.

Prescription NSAIDs, such as celecoxib or diclofenac, pose even more problems. Routine use for pain relief can cause stomach irritation, gastrointestinal bleeding, worsened asthma symptoms, kidney damage, and an increased risk of stroke, heart attack, and blood clots. It's also important to note that the long-term use of either OTC or prescription NSAIDs has been shown to disrupt the composition of the gut microbiome and to contribute to leaky gut syndrome—a condition in which the intestinal lining becomes permeable, allowing toxins and pathogens to escape into the bloodstream. There's no quick fix for leaky gut, and it can lead to a host of health problems throughout the body.

Corticosteroids, on the other hand, are strong inflammation-fighting drugs that are injected into the joint to alleviate pain. Their effects usually last from a few weeks to a few months. While that may sound like the perfect solution to your arthritis pain, these drugs have a dark side, too. Injected corticosteroids can cause facial flushing, insomnia, and high blood sugar. Of more concern, corticosteroid injections can make your arthritis even worse by causing cartilage damage and the death of nearby bone. Because of these side effects and the very real potential to worsen your arthritis, the risks these injections pose likely outweigh the benefits.

And then there are antidepressants like duloxetine (Cymbalta), which was approved by the FDA for use in patients with arthritis of the knee. According to researchers at Tufts Medical Center, about 21 percent of people with arthritis also suffer from depression related to their condition. But like corticosteroids and pain-relieving drugs, these antidepressants carry side effects that can undermine a patient's quality of life. These include difficulty sleeping, headaches, dizziness, blurred vision, constipation, diarrhea, nausea, dry mouth, sweating, tiredness, loss of appetite, weight loss, and a loss of libido or difficulty maintaining an erection. But the problems don't stop there. In rare cases, patients can experience hallucinations, aggression, chronic headaches, confusion, liver problems, or blood in the stool, urine, or vomit. These are serious and frightening side effects.

Surgery is another option for people with severe OA. Joint replacement surgery (technically known as arthroplasty) removes the arthritic and damaged parts of a joint and replaces them with a metal, plastic, or ceramic prosthesis. This prosthesis is designed to mimic the movement of a healthy, normal joint. But, like other conventional joint treatments, it's not risk-free. Complications can include:

- Blood clots
- Dislocation
- Infection
- Injury or damage to the nerves around the replaced joints
- Joint stiffness, weakness, or instability that can lead to fracture

While joint replacement surgery has a fairly good success rate overall, women and older people—the two groups most likely to get arthroplasty—have a higher risk of joint replacement failure. During one study comparing hip replacement in men and women, a group of researchers at the Southern California Permanente Medical Group, Cornell University, and the FDA found that women with an average age of 65 had a 29 percent higher risk of implant failure than men of the same age.

Natural Solutions

If these treatments give you pause or make you feel hopeless, take heart. There are natural ways to proactively protect your joints or even improve your OA symptoms if you're already experiencing joint problems.

Adopting an anti-inflammatory diet that focuses on fruits and vegetables, lean protein, and healthy fats has been found to help prevent OA. When Australian researchers evaluated seven randomized trials, they found that eating an anti-inflammatory diet not only helped the participants lose weight but also reduced inflammatory biomarkers. Both of these benefits are likely to improve OA symptoms. A study published in the *European Journal of Nutrition* reported that an anti-inflammatory diet didn't just foster weight loss; it also improved joint function, pain intensity, depression, anxiety, and overall quality of life in overweight women with knee OA.

Exercise is also important to prevent OA and to maintain joint function if you're already experiencing problems. While most conventional sources recommend moderate aerobic exercise like walking, biking, or swimming, recent investigations suggest that resistance training may be even more beneficial. During one clinical trial, safely lifting heavy weights for 12 weeks increased the participants' isometric knee extensor strength by 37 percent, their isokinetic knee extensor strength by 41 to 47 percent, and their quadriceps and the muscles surrounding their femur bone by 9.8 percent. In this particular study, strengthening the muscles that support knee and hip joints improved pain and function. Strengthening the muscles around the shoulders, elbows, and wrists likely has similar results. One word of caution, though: if you've been diagnosed with OA, it's smart to avoid HIIT workouts since these explosive moves can put further stress on joints.

Joint-Supportive Supplements

What about supplements? Do they really work for OA? Yes! Perhaps the best-known supplemental nutrients for OA are glucosamine and chondroitin. This dynamic duo is naturally produced in the body and supports the structure of your joints. Joint cartilage contains high amounts of both glucosamine and chondroitin. And glucosamine is also found in synovial fluid. But, like many critical compounds our bodies make, production declines with age. Fortunately, long-term supplementation with both glucosamine and chondroitin has been shown to reduce pain and inflammation while improving joint function.

According to a 2018 review of randomized, controlled trials, chondroitin relieved pain and improved joint function while glucosamine improved joint stiffness. These findings aren't surprising since the combination has been shown to also reduce joint-space narrowing. When joint-space narrowing occurs, cartilage no longer keeps the bones a normal distance apart. Over time, this can lead to pain as bone begins to rub against bone.

An earlier review that analyzed 54 studies involving more than 16,000 OA patients found that the combination of glucosamine and chondroitin worked just as well as the OA drug celeboxib to reduce pain, stiffness, and swelling of the knee. Plus, it produced these results without the side effects common to NSAIDs. Just be aware that the benefits glucosamine and chondroitin provide don't come quickly. It can take several months before you see any improvement.

Adding curcumin to the equation, however, can offer faster relief. This powerful anti-inflammatory compound, which is derived from the curry spice turmeric, has been shown to reduce pain just as well as NSAIDs. One 2019 study of nine clinical trials that appeared in the *Annals of the Rheumatic Diseases* found that curcumin was so effective at reducing pain, it allowed participants to reduce their use of NSAIDs and other pain relievers. It also lessened stiffness, improved physical function, and decreased inflammation. In a separate clinical trial involving 50 patients, curcumin reduced pain so much that the participants who took the supplement were 68 percent less likely to reach for a conventional painkiller.

But curcumin does come with a caveat. Standard curcumin supplements are notoriously difficult to absorb because of a lack of solubility. Making matters worse, curcumin is quickly metabolized in the gastrointestinal tract and shuttled out of the body. Because of this, it's critical to look for a high-absorption bioavailable supplement that blends curcumin with turmeric essential oil. Studies show that this combination is nearly seven times more bioavailable compared to typical curcumin supplements. And check the label to ensure it's standardized to supply at least 172 mg of pure curcuminoids, the most active compounds in curcumin.

Extinguish Arthritis Pain with EVOO

While these supplements can be a great jumping off point for managing OA, you can significantly level up your pain relief and dial down inflammation by adding EVOO to your arthritis tool kit. It's also a great way to prevent OA in the first place. And research shows that you can get these results by either supplementing your diet with EVOO or using the oil topically.

For example, in one 2022 study that appeared in the *International Journal of Clinical Practice*, 129 patients with knee OA were assigned to eat either a Mediterranean diet high in EVOO, a low-fat diet, or a standard Western-type diet. Compared to the participants who ate the other two diets, those who ate the

Mediterranean diet experienced a significant reduction in their pain and much improved joint function. As a bonus, they also lost more weight than the people on the low-fat and standard diets.

An earlier preclinical study found that combining physical activity with dietary EVOO also preserved cartilage and protected joints. This suggests that EVOO can be an excellent way to prevent OA if you're at a higher than normal risk of the condition.

Slathering EVOO on affected joints can also help. Anyone with joint pain is likely familiar with those widely advertised tubes of greasy, smelly arthritis creams. But studies show that applying EVOO topically provides even more pain relief than commercial arthritis creams and gels in people with OA of the knee. It's so effective that one study comparing EVOO with the topical drug ketoprofen reported that the oil was just as good as the drug for relieving knee pain. It was also considerably safer since some studies show that routinely using topically applied NSAIDs can result in many of the same side effects as oral NSAIDs, including leaky gut and other gastrointestinal problems.

What is it about EVOO that makes it so beneficial for joints? In a word, oleocanthal. This potent polyphenol has been shown to reduce inflammation by inhibiting prostaglandins and other pro-inflammatory compounds, thus reducing pain. Some research has even compared EVOO to ibuprofen. But unlike ibuprofen, EVOO also reduces the production of inflammatory compounds in the synovial fluid. What's more, research appearing in the journal *Nutrients* has highlighted yet another way EVOO protects joints. According to the 2017 study, the polyphenols in EVOO—especially oleocanthal, oleuropein, and hydroxytyrosol—trigger autophagy. If you remember, autophagy is a natural process the body uses to remove damaged or dysfunctional parts of a cell while leaving the healthy parts intact. But autophagy is compromised in people with OA. By restoring this cellular cleanup process, EVOO can help maintain cartilage health and improve both pain and joint function.

Whether you use EVOO topically or add therapeutic amounts to your diet, studies show that it's one of the most effective ways to protect your joints. From prevention of OA to pain relief, EVOO is an excellent, extremely safe way to keep you on the move.

Shining a Light on Rheumatoid Arthritis

Although OA is the most common form of arthritis, there's another form of the disease that you should be aware of. Like OA, rheumatoid arthritis (RA) causes pain, swelling, and stiffness in the joints. But that's where the similarities end. This is because RA is an inflammatory autoimmune disease that affects many joints at once. Commonly affected joints include the hands, wrists, elbows, shoulders, spine, knees, feet, and jaw. And unlike OA, damage typically appears on both sides of the body. So if a joint is affected in one of your hands or knees, the same joint on the other hand or knee will also be affected.

If you have RA, your body is basically attacking itself. Because the immune system sees the tissue in your joints as foreign, and thus a threat, it sends pro-inflammatory antibodies to attack the joint lining. This causes the lining of joints to become inflamed and, over time, damaged. Eventually, this damage can result in chronic pain, imbalance, and deformity.

Currently, 1.3 million people in the U.S. are affected by RA. Who is more likely to develop this autoimmune condition? People with a genetic predisposition, women—especially those who have never given birth, and those with long-term exposure to airborne environmental contaminants like air pollution or cigarette smoke.

Like OA, there is no cure for RA. That's the bad news. The good news is, you can help manage the disease with many of the same natural strategies used to control the symptoms of OA. These include eating an anti-inflammatory diet and taking curcumin to reduce stiffness and joint swelling. Interesting new research also suggests that the combination of glucosamine and chondroitin can also lessen joint swelling, possibly by improving the gut microbiome.

Several recent studies also point to EVOO as an effective way to reduce RA symptoms. One 2023 cross-sectional trial involving 365 RA patients found that consuming olive oil significantly reduced the inflammatory marker CRP and reduced disease activity.

In another clinical trial of 60 women with RA, applying topical EVOO effectively controlled pain, joint swelling, and RA flare-ups. Based on these findings—and because the oil can safely be used alongside RA medications—adding a daily dose of oral or topical EVOO to your treatment plan may provide better benefits than medication alone, even in those with advanced RA.

CHAPTER 8
Enhance Your Immunity with EVOO

Whether you're trying to sidestep the latest virus or you're looking for protection against a more serious health problem, EVOO has your back. Study after study clearly shows that the polyphenols in EVOO can optimize your defenses by supporting the array of critical immune cells needed to protect against the threats that continually work to undermine your immune response.

As you've seen throughout this book, EVOO doesn't just guard against everyday bacteria and viruses. It also protects against a myriad of chronic conditions. While the monounsaturated fatty acids in olive oil play an important role in preventing or improving degenerative illnesses, research shows that the real secret to EVOO's protective benefits lie in the oil's polyphenols. This is because the polyphenols act directly on your immune cells, optimizing their disease-crushing capabilities. And this could be why EVOO has been shown to lower your risk of an early death. In fact, a large 2022 study by Harvard University researchers found that people consuming high levels of EVOO had a 19 percent lower risk of dying of any cause. More specifically, the researchers found that people consuming robust amounts of EVOO had a 19 percent reduced risk of dying of heart disease, a 17 percent lower risk of dying of cancer, and a 29 percent decreased risk of dying of a neurodegenerative disease like Alzheimer's. But to truly understand how EVOO accomplishes these feats, you need to become better acquainted with how your immune system works.

Immunity 101

Your body's immune system is a complex network of specialized tissues, organs, cells, and chemicals that provide protection against the constant threats you're exposed to from the outside world. When the immune system is running well, it identifies harmful pathogens and works to neutralize them before an infection develops. A strong immune system also guards against chronic illness by seeking out and eliminating any damaged cells it finds in the body.

Accomplishing this search-and-destroy mission requires 24/7 vigilance and not one but three distinct types of immunity. The first is the natural or **innate immunity** you were born with. It's the type of immunity that has been genetically passed down from your parents. The second is **adaptive immunity**, which develops over time as you are exposed to pathogens or immunized against certain diseases. The third is **passive immunity**. This type of immunity is acquired by the transfer of antibodies from another individual, usually from mother to child during birth. Together, these three types of immunity contribute to a strong immune system that ideally protects against a constant and varied assault from bacteria, viruses, and other threats.

While this intricate system works around the clock, it does its job largely unnoticed at a cellular level. Most of the cells in the immune system are white blood cells, also known as leukocytes. There are two basic types of white blood cells, and both are charged with finding disease-causing organisms and destroying them. Here's what each type does:

- **Phagocytes** are white blood cells that gobble up foreign organisms much like a game of PAC-MAN. One of the most common types of phagocyte is the neutrophil, which targets bacteria. Macrophages, another type of phagocyte, function like cellular garbage disposals, ingesting bacteria and cellular debris. Macrophages also produce tumor necrosis factor (TFN), a protein that can kill some types of tumor cells. TFN also mediates inflammation and triggers the creation of new blood vessels.

Specific hormones, collectively known as interleukins, are also triggered by white blood cells. One of these interleukins—interleukin-1—is produced by macrophages after they ingest a foreign microbe. IL-1 triggers fever and fatigue, which assist in killing off many types of bacteria.

- **Lymphocytes**, on the other hand, are produced in your bone marrow. Once created, some lymphocytes stay put and become B-cells. These are considered "smart" immune cells that identify rogue bacteria and viruses that may be lurking in the body. B-cells also remember specific pathogens that have made you sick in the past. Other lymphocytes leave the bone marrow and travel to the thymus, a small gland behind the top of your breastbone, where they turn into T-cells. T-cells are the foot soldiers that destroy the harmful microbes that the B-cells have identified. They are so effective that some types of T-cells are called natural killer (NK) cells. In fact, NK cells are so powerful they can even eradicate certain tumor cells.

When B-cells detect a harmful microbe or toxin—technically known as an antigen—they produce specialized proteins called antibodies that lock onto the invader and disable it. Once disabled, the antigen can be eliminated from the body by the T-cells. Helping the B- and T-cells is something called the complement system. If a harmful microbe makes its way into the bloodstream, a mixture of liquid proteins called complement attacks them, causing them to burst. Complement is made in the liver and works with the antibodies produced by the B-cells.

How Your Habits Undermine a Healthy Immune System

While this cellular army is formidable, it isn't infallible. Many factors can compromise your immunity, including your age, your family history, and your habits. Here are seven ways you're inadvertently weakening your body's ability to protect itself:

1. **You skimp on sleep**. Shortchanging your sleep lowers immune function and reduces the number of NK cells. What's more, chronic sleep deprivation impairs your immune system's surveillance mechanisms and suppresses your immune response.
2. **You live on junk food.** Studies report that eating a diet filled with ultra-processed foods high in sugar and refined carbohydrates triggers chronic inflammation, fosters free-radical damage, and promotes chronically elevated cortisol levels. Together, this increases your susceptibility to colds and other illnesses, boosts your chances of developing food sensitivities, amplifies

gastrointestinal issues, and increases the risk of type 2 diabetes and cancer.

3. **You're a couch potato.** Living a sedentary life can lead to immune dysfunction. According to findings in the journal *Gerontology*, physical inactivity increases your susceptibility to infection and boosts the risk of cancer, cardiovascular disease, and autoimmune disorders.
4. **You're exposed to cigarette smoke**. Exposure to tobacco smoke increases the risk of developing cancer, cardiovascular disease, and respiratory disorders. That's not surprising since research in the journal *Oncotarget* shows that smokers have compromised B- and T-cells.
5. **You're constantly stressed out.** Chronic stress lowers your NK cell count and diminishes the activity of macrophages and other types of T-cells. This is why it's not uncommon to come down with a virus after a period of prolonged stress.
6. **You're a "glass half empty" type of person.** Clinical trials have found that how you view the world has a direct impact on your immune response. One study of 220 adults that appeared in the journal *Brain, Behavior, and Immunity* found that those with a negative attitude had higher inflammatory biomarkers.

7. **You're a loner.** Research shows that the less you interact with others, the more prone you are to getting sick. According to one 2021 study, loneliness alters the immune system, setting the stage for chronic inflammation while also reducing immune cell activity and antibody response.

Aging, Immunity, and EVOO

When we are young, most of us have a robust immune system. But once we hit the ripe old age of 65, our defenses aren't as efficient as they once were. That may be why many seniors find they are more vulnerable to developing chronic diseases and infections—and why the elderly often have a poor response to treatments and vaccinations. These age-related changes to our immune system are known among researchers as **immunosenescence**. A lifetime of wear and tear contributes to these age-related changes. Plus, exposure to environmental contaminants over the years can further undermine the immune system. While we can't stop the clock, we can slow down the deterioration of the immune system. And one of the easiest ways to do this is with EVOO.

Research out of Spain shows that EVOO not only targets the hallmarks of aging like mitochondrial dysfunction and the shortening of our telomeres. It also modulates the immune system. This, in turn, helps prevent out-of-control inflammation that can undermine a healthy immune response as we grow older. Because of their findings, the Spanish scientists suggest that swapping out other types of dietary fat for polyphenol-rich EVOO can restore immune function to that of our considerably younger selves.

The Immune-Supportive Secrets of EVOO

EVOO works in multiple ways to optimize the immune system, and they all revolve around its high polyphenol content. Because polyphenols have powerful antioxidant and anti-inflammatory activity, they are able to limit the oxidative stress and chronic inflammation that has been linked to a weakened immune system and most chronic diseases. The polyphenols in EVOO have also been shown to possess a wide range of properties that enhance the oil's immune-protective reputation. These include EVOO's anticancer, antidiabetic, antifungal, antihypertensive, anti-inflammatory, antimicrobial, antioxidant, antiviral, cardioprotective, gastroprotective, neuroprotective, and pain-relieving properties. Talk about multitasking! Few foods can provide this much protection.

Three particular polyphenols—oleuropein, hydroxytyrosol, and tyrosol—have captured the focus of most research linking EVOO to enhanced immunity. Several studies show that oleuropein is a powerful antiviral, and at least one of these studies reports significant protection against respiratory infections like the respiratory syncytial virus (RSV) and the parainfluenza virus type 3. It also has a beneficial impact on hepatitis B. Other research suggests that hydroxytyrosol could be effective against seasonal flu. And a five-minute room-temperature test showed that hydroxytyrosol and tyrosol decreased the activity of Listeria monocytogenes, a type of bacteria that can cause serious food poisoning.

Most of this immune-boosting activity happens on a cellular level. For instance, a 2018 study out of Italy found that oleuropein modifies the way the immune system responded to harmful pathogens by increasing the production of interferon-gamma—a type of immune cell that activates macrophages—as well as NK cells and another kind of T-cell called CD8+. And when paired with hydroxytyrosol, this powerful polyphenol helps keep out-of-control inflammation in check by acting directly on inflammation-stoking cytokines like interleukin-1 or interleukin-6.

Research conducted in 2022 reports that hydroxytyrosol can also strengthen a weakened immune system by boosting the activity of T-cells while enhancing the activity of superoxide dismutase (SOD) and glutathione—two of the body's most important antioxidants. One reason hydroxytyrosol is so effective is because it increases immunity in the gastrointestinal system—and that's hugely important since at least 70 percent of your immune system is found in your gut.

Since so much of the immune system is located in the mucosal lining of the gut, researchers have started looking at how the microbiome—the collection of microbes in your large intestine—impact immunity. One 2021 study in the journal *Nutrition Reviews* reports that EVOO reduces harmful bacteria in the gut while stimulating the growth of beneficial bacteria. At the same time, the researchers noted that EVOO increases the production of short-chain fatty acids that help regulate inflammation and the immune response. These findings build on earlier research showing that a Mediterranean diet high in EVOO increases one particular type of beneficial bacteria known as bacteroides that have strong anti-inflammatory capabilities.

These three super polyphenols aren't the only beneficial compounds in EVOO. Oleocanthal also plays a role in supporting a healthy immune response. This was first observed nearly two decades ago by biologist Gary Beauchamp, who now serves as the director emeritus of the Monell Chemical Senses Center in Philadelphia. While in Sicily, he experienced a ticklish peppery sensation in the back of his throat after tasting some EVOO. He noticed that it was very similar to the sensation he had during his research when swallowing liquid forms of aspirin and ibuprofen. Since Beauchamp's first observation, studies have found that oleocanthal not only triggers the same sensation created by over-the-counter NSAIDs; it also inhibits the COX-1 and COX-2 enzymes that cause pain and inflammation, acting in much the same way these drugs do.

Another polyphenol shown to influence the immune system is oleacein. Studies have found that oleacein has antioxidant, anti-inflammatory, and anticancer activity. It also kick-starts apoptosis, the programmed cell death that helps prevent the spread of cancer in the body. But one of oleacein's most important benefits is its ability to modulate the immune response, essentially helping to ensure that the immune system doesn't overreact to something it sees as a threat. And that's a real boon for anyone with an autoimmune disease.

EVOO and Autoimmunity

It's estimated that between 24 and 50 million Americans are currently afflicted by some type of autoimmune disease, such as celiac disease, lupus, inflammatory bowel disease, or rheumatoid arthritis. All of these conditions have one thing in common: an overactive immune response that can't tell the difference between a harmful pathogen and the body's own tissues. As a result, the immune system goes into overdrive and attacks healthy tissue by mistake.

Research shows that the polyphenols in EVOO reduced bacterial toxins while also minimizing oxidative damage in a model of multiple sclerosis. And another study in the Journal of Nutritional Biochemistry reports that olive oil reduced both acute and chronic inflammation in rheumatoid arthritis.

A diet high in oleocanthal-rich EVOO has also been shown to improve the immune response and physiological damage that affects those with lupus. Lupus is a serious long-term autoimmune disease that can cause chronic inflammation in the skin, organs, and various other parts of the body. People with this condition experience rashes, anemia, high blood pressure, kidney problems, joint pain, and endothelial dysfunction. But oleocanthal has been shown to reduce the levels of the compounds that spark inflammation. As a result, oleocanthal-rich EVOO improves both the symptoms and progression of the disease.

Whether you're living with an autoimmune disease, have a higher than average risk of developing a chronic condition, or simply want to guard against whatever bug happens to be going around, EVOO can help optimize your defenses. But to get these medicinal benefits, make sure that you choose the right EVOO. In the next chapter, we'll take a deep dive into what you should look for.

CHAPTER 9
How to Choose and Use EVOO

It's abundantly clear that EVOO is one of the foundational keys to good health and longevity. The problem is, purchasing a high-quality oil is sometimes easier said than done. After all, when it's time to choose, you're often faced with supermarket shelves filled with bottles of olive oil from a wide array of countries. How do you know which ones are authentic and which ones boast the highest polyphenol levels? The truth is, the best EVOO starts with the olives and how they are processed.

Harvesting and Producing the Best Olive Oil

Traditionally, olives were hand-picked directly from the branches and dropped into baskets or nets—and it's a method still used by small artisanal olive oil producers today. This method allows growers to harvest olives as gently as possible when they are young and green to minimize damage and maximize the polyphenols. As a result, it's the first step in producing the highest-quality, most nutritious olive oil. The problem is, handpicking olives is extremely labor-intensive. This makes it the least efficient and the most expensive way to harvest olives.

In an effort to increase the harvest and cut costs, another technique known as bacchiatura is used to beat the olive branches with sticks to make the olives fall into nets placed on the ground. While this method originally used human labor to beat the olive trees, today's larger growers use automated methods to either shake or comb the olives from their branches. During shaking, mechanical arms wrap around the trunk or branches of the olive tree and shake the tree to encourage the fruit to fall. Combing, on the other hand, uses special tools to separate the olives from the branches. The olives are then collected in nets that are attached under the trees. These industrialized methods are approximately four times faster than handpicking olives, which means the olives can move very quickly from harvest to pressing.

Extracting the oil from the olives is a complex process. Once the fruit has been harvested, it is prone to oxidation. Because of this, the olives are immediately transported to the mill where they are graded and washed. For olive oil producers using traditional pressing methods, the olives are then crushed with large stone grinding plates and the resulting mash is placed on porous straw or burlap disks. These mats are then stacked and slowly pressed to extract the oil. The oil is separated from the runoff and filtered (although some producers leave the oil unfiltered) before being bottled. The entire process is done on the estate where the olives are grown. This artisanal approach produces cold-pressed polyphenol-rich EVOO of the highest quality. But because this process is so labor-intensive, only limited quantities can be produced.

Today's large producers, on the other hand, use electronically controlled milling equipment to crush vast amounts of olives quickly. Because this limits the fruit's exposure to oxygen, this type of milling prevents oxidation and helps preserve the healthful compounds in the olives. The mash is then kneaded using a machine called a malaxer to break up the bonds that formed between the water and the oil during the crushing process.

Instead of pressing the mash to extract the oil, modern olive processing uses a centrifuge that spins very fast to separate the oil from the water and pulp. Once extracted, the oil is filtered and decanted into large steel containers to await bottling. While ancient olive growers wouldn't recognize these high-tech methods, the olives are never subjected to heat, and care is taken to preserve both the fruit's polyphenolic compounds and the finished oil's sensory properties. As a result, these modern methods can produce a high-quality cold-pressed EVOO that is bitter, fruity, pungent, and free of any defects.

Once the first press has been completed, the remaining mash is then pressed again. But because the mash now contains much less oil, heat is applied to coax any remaining oil from the fruit. This oil is often called "light" olive oil—not because it contains fewer calories but because it has a lighter taste and considerably fewer polyphenols.

After two pressings, most of the oil has been extracted, but a small amount remains. A third pressing uses solvents like hexane to extract this remaining oil. The problem is, this oil—known as lampante—isn't edible and must be refined with neutralizing compounds as well as bleaching and deodorizing chemicals. The resulting oil is sold as "pure olive oil" or simply "olive oil." This type of processing creates a highly compromised version of the real deal that has been stripped of most of its healthful properties.

Making the Grade

All olive oil is graded based on how it was processed and the finished product's acidity. There are four grades of olive oil.

Extra virgin olive oil is extracted solely by mechanical means without using heat or solvents. This protects the nutrients in the olives. According to international standards, EVOO is free of defects and flavor flaws and has an excellent odor. It is also required to have a free fatty acid content that is not more 0.8 percent. EVOO produced in California is subject to even stricter requirements as it can't have an acidity higher than 0.5 percent. True EVOO accounts for less than 10 percent of all olive oil in many countries that produce the oil.

Like EVOO, **virgin olive oil** is processed using mechanical means without the use of heat or solvents. However, it's allowed acidity is higher—up to 2 percent.

It's also allowed to have some minor defects while maintaining a good flavor. This indicates that the oil has a relatively high polyphenol content, but it's not as nutritious as EVOO.

Refined olive oil means that the oil has undergone additional processing to neutralize any defects in taste, aroma, or acidity. Although it has an acidity of no more than 0.3 percent, it is flavorless and odorless, indicating that it's a lower-quality oil with only trace amounts of polyphenols. Any nutrients contained in refined olive oil typically come from small amounts of EVOO that are added to the oil.

Refined olive pomace oil is the lowest grade of olive oil. Obtained from the last pressing, crude pomace oil is unfit for human consumption and must be refined using solvents and heat during the extraction and refining processes to make it safe and edible. Refined olive pomace oil isn't typically sold in supermarkets but is often used in restaurant kitchens for frying since it lacks flavor and has a relatively high smoke point.

Fraud Alert!

You might assume that once you know the different grades of olive oil, it would be pretty straightforward to find a healthful high-quality product at your local supermarket. Unfortunately, that's not always the case. Fraud is rampant when it comes to olive oil. According to a 2011 study conducted at the University of California,

Davis, nearly three-quarters of all oils sold as EVOO failed to meet internationally accepted standards. These findings rocked the olive oil industry and shocked foodies around the world. And yet, things haven't gotten any better in the ensuing years. In fact, when Danish researchers sampled 35 different brands of EVOO in 2017, only 6 were found to be authentic EVOO.

Between 2016 and 2019, the Joint Research Centre—which is the internal scientific department of the European Commission—gathered data about potential fraud. They identified 32 cases of fake or adulterated EVOO globally. Most were due to mislabeling or the substitution or dilution of olive oil with cheaper, inferior oils. One crime ring was even accused of coloring low-quality soy or canola oil with industrial chlorophyll and flavoring it with beta-carotene before passing it off as EVOO.

Despite all of this bait and switch, it's still possible to purchase a high-quality EVOO that's brimming with health benefits. But because regulatory agencies in Europe and the United States don't routinely test olive oil for authenticity, uncovering the fakes and frauds comes down to being an educated consumer.

How to Pick the Healthiest Olive Oil

Since you can't rely on government agencies to screen your EVOO, it's basically up to you. But with so many options on store shelves, where should you start and what should you look for? Fortunately, there are some tips to help you choose the best.

The best of the best EVOO often lists its acidity level, the type of olive it's made from, the harvest date, and the country of origin. These oils are typically bottled in black, dark-brown, or opaque white glass bottles. Some are bottled in lighter glass and packaged in an outer cardboard box to protect the oil's health benefits. But these premium EVOOs don't come cheap. A 16-ounce bottle can start at $25 and go up from there. Are they worth it? Absolutely!

But high price doesn't necessarily guarantee high quality. Luckily, there are organizations that independently certify olive oils to help ensure you're getting a healthful, high-quality product. For instance, the North American Olive Oil Association (NAOOA) provides a quality-seal program that tests and verifies the authenticity and purity of a wide range of olive oils. To obtain this certification, association members agree to have their oils tested twice per year to ensure that they meet or exceed International Olive Council standards. Samples are obtained from oils purchased in the general marketplace, and testing includes both sensory (taste and smell) and chemical tests.

NAOOA isn't the only regulating body to certify olive oil. The California Olive Oil Council (COOC) also has a certification program that evaluates EVOO for quality using sensory tests and some chemical tests. While samples are provided by the olive oil producers themselves, the COOC seal is exclusively limited to EVOO.

You may be able to find an affordable option, even without certification. Armed with some knowledge, you can unearth good-quality polyphenol-rich EVOO in a store near you.

- Look for dark, opaque bottles or metallic containers that don't expose the oil to sunlight. This is important since sunlight can quickly degrade the polyphenols in EVOO.
- Look for the harvest date, which is included on labels by some top olive oil producers. If that's not present, look for the "best by" date. Try to buy an oil with a date as far into the future as possible. This suggests a higher level of polyphenols.
- Look for a low fatty acid content. The acidity must be less than 0.8 percent for a high-quality EVOO produced in Europe and 0.5 percent for an EVOO produced in California.
- If purchasing EVOO from a country in the EU, look for an organic seal and a DOP (protected designation of origin) or PGI (protected geographical indication) marking. These ensure that the oil meets European Union standards for EVOO.
- Choose a smaller bottle (think 16.9 ounces max). Once you open the bottle, your EVOO will immediately begin to oxidize and degrade, so it's wise to opt for a size that you can consume within a month.

Become an Olive Oil Sommelier!

Since there are no standards for labeling, choosing a bottle of EVOO in the supermarket can be hit or miss, even if you know what to look for. But there's one simple trick that can help you figure out if your EVOO is authentic and packed with those good-for-you polyphenols—the taste test.

- Pour approximately 2 tablespoons of the oil into a small, round glass (a shot glass works well).
- While cupping the glass with one hand, cover the top with the other hand to trap the aroma inside. Move the glass in a circular motion.
- Uncover the glass and take a deep whiff of the oil. It should have a strong, fresh scent of grass fruit, or a peppery vegetable like arugula. This is a good indication that the oil is truly extra virgin. If it smells like Play-Doh, crayons, or old walnuts, the oil is rancid.
- The final step is to taste the oil, a process that's much like tasting wine. Take a small sip but don't swallow. With clenched teeth and open lips, inhale through your mouth. Close your lips and swish the oil around in your mouth. You may taste fruity or green notes as you swirl the oil. Finally, swallow the oil. True EVOO will leave a peppery sensation at the back of your throat. High-polyphenol

EVOO should also give you a tickle in your throat and could likely produce a cough or two.

The Fridge-Test Fallacy

Maybe you've heard that the best way to test the authenticity of EVOO is to put it in the fridge. If it solidifies, it's the genuine article—or at least that's what proponents say. The only problem is that, according to the University of California, Davis Olive Center, it's not an accurate way to verify your EVOO. It may not even tell you if your oil is actually made of olives!

These conclusions were based on a study in which the researchers refrigerated seven samples of different oils. Two were unrefined EVOO, one was a refined olive oil, and others included canola oil, safflower oil, and two oil blends. Though some of the oils had mild congealing at the bottom of the bottles after being refrigerated for 60 hours, none solidified completely. Even after 180 hours, none of the samples fully solidified.

Drinking EVOO Medicinally

To get the most health benefits from your bottle of high-polyphenol EVOO, drink a small amount daily. Several studies show that consuming just 25 mL, which is about 2 tablespoons, of EVOO has a protective effect against oxidative damage, chronic inflammation, atherosclerosis, and type 2 diabetes. That may be why people living in Mediterranean countries typically enjoy such robust health. In fact, Spaniards and Italians typically consume a little more than 2 tablespoons each day. And Greeks, who have the highest intake in the world, drink nearly 5 tablespoons each day!

If 2 tablespoons seems like a lot all at once, start slowly with 1 teaspoon and gradually work your way up to the full dose. You can also boost your intake by drizzling it on salads, vegetables, or dips like hummus or baba ghanoush (a delicious Lebanese eggplant dip). If drinking EVOO straight upsets your stomach, consider taking it with a meal as you would most dietary supplements.

Cooking with EVOO

What about swapping out your regular cooking oil with EVOO? Is it even safe? The misconception that EVOO isn't safe to cook with originated with the mistaken assumption about the oil's "smoke point." Smoke point is the temperature at which an oil begins to break down and smoke. Yet, people in Mediterranean countries have been safely cooking and baking with EVOO for centuries. And modern research confirms that the oil is extremely stable up to 464°F. This means that EVOO is ideal for all types of cooking—including deep-frying.

How does EVOO's safety compare to other common cooking oils? Research published in 2018 found that compared to canola oil, grapeseed oil, and rice bran oil, EVOO produces the lowest levels of polar compounds, making it the safest and most stable oil to cook with. Canola, grapeseed, and rice bran oils, on the other hand were relatively unstable and produced high levels of polar compounds. That matters since high levels of polar compounds—which are formed when these oils are exposed to high heat—have been linked to Alzheimer's and Parkinson's diseases.

But smoke point isn't the only misconception that keeps people from cooking with EVOO. Some people claim that all the health benefits are lost when the oil is heated. This is due to the common belief that heat degrades or destroys nutrients, including the polyphenols in EVOO. Yet, this too has been shown to be false. According to a 2022 study by the University of Barcelona that appeared in the journal *Trends in Food Science & Technology*, EVOO is less prone to oxidation than other monounsaturated cooking oils like peanut or canola oil. That helps preserve the beneficial fatty acids and vitamins in EVOO. The Spanish researchers also found that the antioxidants in the oil were transferred to food during cooking. Plus, the polyphenols in EVOO prevent the formation of acrylamide, a carcinogen that is formed when foods are cooked at high heat (for instance, baking, frying, grilling, or roasting).

These results build on earlier research by the same scientists that found that EVOO retains significant nutrient levels during cooking. During their study, the researchers heated the EVOO and other common cooking oils to temperatures between 258°F and 338°F. While the antioxidant-rich polyphenol content of the EVOO decreased by 40 percent at 258°F and by 75 percent at 338°F, it still contained 500 percent more antioxidants than other oils.

These findings mean that, although you will lose some health benefits when you cook with EVOO, you'll still get considerably more antioxidants than you would if you cooked with other oils—even healthy oils like avocado or coconut. And those nutrients are transferred to the food you're cooking. This was seen in a 2015 study out of Mexico that reported that potatoes fried in EVOO contained more phenols and antioxidants than potatoes boiled in water.

Level Up With Olive Leaf

While cooking with EVOO—and even drinking it—are excellent ways to tap into this golden elixir's many health properties, you can obtain even more health benefits by adding an olive leaf extract supplement. This is because studies show that the leaves from the humble olive tree provide a concentrated source of the same beneficial bioactives found in EVOO—especially oleuropein, hydroxytyrosol, and oleanolic acid. Plus, the leaves are a good source of two other powerful free radical fighters—maslinic acid and vitamin E. Research reports that the compounds in olive leaf extract don't just boast powerful antioxidant properties, they also provide a wealth of antimicrobial, antiviral, and anti-inflammatory activity. As a result, supplementation can help to support optimal cardiovascular, digestive, immune, metabolic, and neurological health. But to get all these health benefits, opt for a supplement that provides at least 500 mg of a full spectrum olive leaf extract and take it once or twice daily. Pairing EVOO with a high-quality olive leaf extract can help ensure you're getting a consistent, high potency dose of polyphenols for better health every day.

But even though these studies prove that EVOO is the best oil for most types of cooking, don't use it in dishes that are cooked in the microwave. Microwaving increases the oil's acidity and levels of a toxin called acrolein. Acrolein is a member of the aldehyde family, and it's a strong irritant that triggers inflammation. What's more, this form of cooking decreases the polyphenols in EVOO more than panfrying.

With all the health benefits you'll enjoy by cooking with EVOO, you might be wondering if all your food will end up tasting like the oil. Even though EVOO has a robust flavor when raw, heating destroys the delicate flavor compounds in the oil, thus reducing its taste significantly. This means that EVOO won't mask the flavor of the foods cooked in the oil.

Whether consumed raw or cooked, incorporating EVOO into your daily life can provide a wealth of health benefits thanks to its powerful antioxidant and anti-inflammatory qualities. And because the polyphenols in EVOO can target a variety of chronic conditions, it's a great way to prevent or even improve many of the health problems that plague society today. And when you add this remarkable oil to an already healthy diet and lifestyle, you'll discover one of the easiest and tastiest ways to level up your health and well-being.

"Published studies show that no other food comes close to Extra Virgin Olive Oil for the prevention and treatment of chronic disease."

Mary M. Flynn, PhD, RD, LDN

Associate Professor of Medicine (Clinical), Brown University

Founder of The Olive Oil Health Initiative, Miriam Hospital

RESOURCES

To get all the health benefits EVOO has to offer, seek out an oil that has low acidity and provides high polyphenol levels. This is considered medicinal-quality olive oil.

What's more, a high-quality EVOO should consist of 55 to 85 percent oleic acid, which is an omega-9 fatty acid (see Chapter 2). These omega-9s not only provide health benefits, they also help prevent the oxidation and degradation of the oil itself. While other healthy oils (think avocado, macadamia, and pecan) also boast omega-9s, they have few if any polyphenols. The combination of polyphenols and omega-9s give EVOO a higher nutritional value and longer shelf life than oils with a lower oleic acid content.

Premium Extra Virgin Olive Oils

Though admittedly expensive, the olive oils on this list contain the highest polyphenol levels, which is why they are among the olive oils I use. For me, these EVOOs are a part of the very best "medicines" in my personal health kit.

- **kyoord.** This premium brand of high-phenolic EVOO was founded by Dr. Limor Goren, a cancer researcher with a PhD in molecular biology. Made in Corfu, Greece, kyoord EVOO is extremely rich in polyphenols (903 mg/kg), most notably oleocanthal and oleacein. kyoord EVOO starts with unripe green olives that are hand-harvested from the company's small family farm early in the season. They are then pressed within hours to produce EVOO with extremely low acidity. Each of the company's oils is analyzed and certified by the World Olive Center for Health in Athens for its polyphenol content.
- **Kosterina.** Cold-pressed in small batches, this EVOO is created from a single blend of early-harvest Koroneiki olives grown in southern Greece. Their original EVOO contains high levels of polyphenols, measuring 570 mg/kg, as reported by a third-party chemical analysis as soon as the harvest is complete each year. In addition, Kosterina's EVOO is certified organic with an acidity level of 0.17 percent.
- **Liokareas.** This olive estate has been pressing olive oil for more than five generations. Their Rx High Polyphenol Extra Virgin Olive Oil (HPEVOO) is notably abundant in polyphenols, especially

oleocanthal. Using old-world methods to harvest the olives, Liokareas EVOO is pressed on the company's family-owned orchard in the foothills of Kalamata in southern Greece. In 2023, their HPEVOO won gold at Spain's World's Best Healthy Extra Virgin Olive Oil Contest for its healthy composition of fatty acids, oleocanthal, and biophenols.

Good-Quality Extra Virgin Olive Oils

Although the following oils have lower polyphenol levels, they still provide a wealth of health benefits, but at a more reasonable price point.

- **Bari.** With roots back to 1936, Bari is one of the oldest olive oil companies in the United States. Many of the olives used to create its cold-pressed EVOO are grown on the company's family-run olive groves. Other olives are sourced from local family farms to ensure quality and freshness. Located in California's San Joaquin Valley, Bari is a winner of numerous awards, including a gold medal at the prestigious Los Angeles International Olive Oil Competition.
- **Bellucci.** This Italian EVOO is created by a collective of small family-owned olive groves that harvest olives by hand using

traditional methods. Each type of EVOO it sells lists the varieties of olives used to make the oil. What's more, each batch of Bellucci EVOO is traced from tree to bottle to ensure quality and potency. Bellucci's EVOO has also earned a silver medal at the Los Angeles International Olive Oil Competition.

- **California Olive Ranch.** The flagship EVOO produced by California Olive Ranch is pressed from olives grown exclusively in California. Each bottle also features the company's smart labeling system, which allows consumers to scan a QR code that takes them to a website where they can learn about the origins of the product, including selected chemical data on the quality and healthfulness of the oil.
- **García de la Cruz**. This company was founded in 1872 by Adelaida Fernandez-Cuellar, in an era when it was uncommon for women to own businesses. Today, this family-run company located in Montes de Toledo, Spain, cultivates a variety of olives—all 100 percent organically grown—and labels each bottle with both the harvest date and the "best by" date. Their EVOO is certified by the North American Olive Oil Association and has won multiple awards from various competitions in Los Angeles, New York, and Japan.

- **Morocco Gold**. The EVOO from Morocco Gold comes from olive groves located in the foothills of Morocco's Atlas Mountains. The oil is made from a single source—Picholine Marocaine olives—which are selected early in the season, handpicked, and cold-pressed within 24 hours of harvest. Because Picholine olives are naturally high in antioxidants, this EVOO contains a polyphenol level of 644 mg/kg. At 0.2 percent, it's also quite low in acidity.

REFERENCES

Introduction

Clodoveo ML, Camposeo S, De Gennaro B, et al. In the ancient world, virgin olive oil was called "liquid gold" by Homer and "the great healer" by Hippocrates. Why has this mythic image been forgotten? *Food Research International.* 2014;62:1062–8.

Frankel EN, Mailer RJ, Wang SC, et al. Evaluation of extra-virgin olive oil sold in California. UC Davis Olive Center at the Robert Mondavi Institute. 2011. http://vrisi36.com/wp-content/uploads/UCDavis-Report.pdf.

Chapter 1: Olive Oil Through the Ages

Ali SA, Parveen N, Ali AS. Links between the Prophet Muhammad (PBUH) recommended foods and disease management: A review in the light of modern superfoods. *International Journal of Health Sciences* (Qassim). 2018;12(2):61–9.

Caramia G. L'olio extra vergine d'oliva. Dalla leggenda al razionale scientifico degli aspetti nutraceutici [Virgin olive oil. From legend to scientific knowledge of the nutraceutical aspects]. *La Pediatria Medica e Chirurgica.* 2006;28(1–3):9–23.

Chaiyana W, Leelapornpisid P, Prongpradist R, et al. Enhancement of antioxidant and skin moisturizing effects of olive oil by incorporation into microemulsions. Nanomaterials and Nanotechnology. 2016;6:1–8.

Curry A. Ancient Roman vacationers consumed gobs of olive oil and fish, volcano victims reveal. *Science.* 2021.

Kapellakis IE. Olive oil history, production and by-product management. Reviews in Environmental Science and Bio/Technology. 2008;7(1):1–26.

Kaur CD, Saraf S. In vitro sun protection factor determination of herbal oils used in cosmetics. *Pharmacognosy Research.* 2010;2(1):22–5.

Lin TK, Zhong L, Santiago JL. Anti-inflammatory and skin barrier repair effects of topical application of some plant oils. *International Journal of Molecular Science.* 2017;19(1):70.

Marquer L, Otto T, Arous EB, et al. The first use of olives in Africa around 100,000 years ago. *Nature Plants.* 2022;8:204–8.

Olive oil consumption in the United States from 2000 to 2021. Statista. https://www.statista.com/statistics/288368/olive-oil-consumption-united-states/

Vossen P. Olive oil: history, production, and characteristics of the world's classic oils. *HortScience.* 2007;42(5):1093–100.

Yapijakis C. Hipppocrates of Kos, the father of clinical medicine, and Asclepiades of Bithynim, the father of molecular medicine. In Vivo. 2009;23(4):507–14.

Chapter 2: What Makes Olive Oil So Darn Healthy?

Abdallah IM, Al-Shami KM, Yang E, et al. Oleuropein-rich olive leaf extract attenuates neuroinflammation in the Alzheimer's disease mouse model. *ACS Chemical Neuroscience.* 2022;13(7):1002–13.

Al Rihani SB, Darakjian LI, Kaddoumi A. Oleocanthal-rich extra-virgin olive oil restores the blood-brain barrier function through NLRP3 inflammasome inhibition simultaneously with autophagy induction in TgSwDI mice. *ACS Chemical Neuroscience.* 2019;10(8):3543–54.

Arangia A, Marino Y, Impellizzeri D, et al. Hydroxytyrosol and its potential uses on intestinal and gastrointestinal disease. *International Journal of Molecular Sciences.* 2023;24:3111.

Barbaro B, Toietta G, Maggio R, et al. Effects of the olive-derived polyphenol oleuropein on human health. *International Journal of Molecular Science.* 2014;15:18508–24.

Babu S, Jayaraman S. An update on β-sitosterol: A potential herbal nutraceutical for diabetic management. *Biomedicine & Pharmacotherapy.* 2020;131:110702.

Berges RR, Kassen A, Senge T. Treatment of symptomatic benign prostatic hyperplasia with beta-sitosterol: an 18-month follow-up. *BJU International.* 2000;85(7):842–6.

Binukumar B, Mathew A. Dietary fat and risk of breast cancer. *World Journal of Surgical Oncology.* 2005;3:45.

Boskou D, Blekas G, Tsimidou M. Olive Oil Composition. Editor(s): Dimitrios Boskou. Olive Oil (Second Edition). AOCS Press. 2006;41–72.

Chen MN, Lin CC, Liu CF. Efficacy of phytoestrogens for menopausal symptoms: a meta-analysis and systematic review. *Climacteric.* 2015;18(2):260–9.

Fistonić I, Situm M, Bulat V, et al. Olive oil biophenols and women's health. *Medicinski Glasnik (Zenica).* 2012;9(1):1–9.

Florence TM. The role of free radicals in disease. *Australian & New Zealand Journal of Ophthalmology.* 1995;23(1):3–7.

Gorzynik-Debicka M, Przychodzen P, Cappello F, et al. Potential health benefits of olive oil and plant polyphenols. *International Journal of Molecular Science.* 2018;19(3):686.

Guasch M, Liu G, Li Y, et al. Olive oil consumption and risk of cardiovascular disease. *Circulation.* 2020;141:AP509.

Guasch-Ferré M, Hu FB, Martinez-Gonzalez MA, et al. Olive oil intake and risk of cardiovascular disease and mortality in the PREDIMED study. *BMC Medicine.* 2014;12:78.

Guasch-Ferré M, Li Y, Willett W, et al. Consumption of olive oil and risk of total and cause-specific mortality among U.S. adults. *Journal of American College of Cardiology.* 2022;79(2): 101–12.

Halder M, Petsophonsakul P, Akbulut AC, et al. Vitamin K: double bonds beyond coagulation insights into differences between vitamin K1 and K2 in health and disease. *International Journal of Molecular Science.* 2019;20(4):896.

Hassan Sakar E, Gharby S. Olive Oil: Extraction Technology, Chemical Composition, and Enrichment Using Natural Additives. *Olive Cultivation.* 2022.

Huang ZR, Lin YK, Fang JY. Biological and pharmacological activities of squalene and related compounds: potential uses in cosmetic dermatology. *Molecules.* 2009;14(1):540–54.

Jimenez-Lopez C, Carpena M, Lourenço-Lopes C, et al. Bioactive compounds and quality of extra virgin olive oil. *Foods.* 2020;9(8):1014.

Kien CL, Bunn JY, Tompkins CL, et al. Substituting dietary monounsaturated fat for saturated fat is associated with increased daily physical activity and resting energy expenditure and with changes in mood. *American Journal of Clinical Nutrition.* 2013;97(4):689–97.

Kim TH, Jung JW, Ha BG, et al. The effects of luteolin on osteoclast differentiation, function in vitro and ovariectomy-induced bone loss. *The Journal of Nutritional Biochemistry.* 2011;22(1): 8–15.

Kris-Etherton PM. AHA science advisory: monounsaturated fatty acids and risk of cardiovascular disease. *Journal of Nutrition.* 1999;129(12):2280–4.

Kwon SY, Massey K, Watson MA, et al. Oxidised metabolites of the omega-6 fatty acid linoleic acid activate dFOXO. *Life Science Alliance.* 2020;3(2):e201900356.

Liu M, Wallmon A, Olsson-Mortlock C, Wallin R, et al. Mixed tocopherols inhibit platelet aggregation in humans:

potential mechanisms. *American Journal of Clinical Nutrition.* 2003;77(3):700–6.

Lukic M, Lukic I, Moslavac T. Sterols and triterpene diols in virgin olive oil: a comprehensive review on their properties and significance, with a special emphasis on the influence of variety and ripening degree. *Horticulture.* 2021;7:493.

Markovic AK, Toric J, Barbaric M, et al. Hydroxytyrosol, tyrosol and derivatives and their potential effects on human health. *Molecules.* 2019;24:2001.

Martirosyan D, Ashoori MR, Serani A, et al. Assessment of squalene effect on antioxidant enzymes and free radicals in patients with type 2 diabetes mellitus. *Bioactive Compounds in Health and Disease.* 2022;5(11):236–50.

Martinez L, Ros G, Nieto G. Hydroxytyrosol: health benefits and use as functional ingredient in meat. *Medicines.* 2018;5:13.

Mateos R, Sarria B, Bravo L. Nutritional and other health properties of olive pomace oil. *Critical Reviews in Food Science and Nutrition.* 2020;60(20):3506–21.

Menezes RCR, Peres, KK, Costa-Valle MT, et al. Oral administration of oleuropein and olive leaf extract has cardioprotective effects in rodents: A systematic review. Revista Portuguesa de Cardiologia. 2022;41(2):167–75.

Mirmiran P, Houshialsadat Z, Bahadoran Z, et al. Association of dietary fatty acids and the incidence risk of cardiovascular disease in adults: the Tehran Lipid and Glucose Prospective Study. *BMC Public Health.* 2020;20:1743.

Miró-Casas E, Covas M-I, Fitó M, et al. Tyrosol and hydroxytyrosol are absorbed from moderate and sustained doses of virgin olive oil in humans. *European Journal of Clinical Nutrition.* 2003;57(1):186–90.

Paunescu AC, Ayotte P, Dewailly E, et al. Saturated and monounsaturated fatty acid status is associated with bone strength estimated by calcaneal ultrasonography in Inuit women from Nunavik (Canada): a cross-sectional study. *Journal of Nutrition, Health & Aging*. 2014;18(7):663–71.

Phylloquinone biosynthesis and engineering in plants. United States Department of Agriculture/University of Nebraska. 2013. https://reeis.usda.gov/web/crisprojectpages/0215789-phylloquinone-biosynthesis-and-engineering-in-plants.html.

Raposio E, Grieco MP, Caleffi E. Evaluation of plasma oxidative stress, with or without antioxidant supplementation, in superficial partial thickness burn patients: a pilot study. *Journal of Plastic Surgery and Hand Surgery*. 2017;51(6):393–8.

Richman EL, Kenfield SA, Chavarro JE, et al. Fat intake after diagnosis and risk of lethal prostate cancer and all-cause mortality. *JAMA Internal Medicine*. 2013;173(14):1318–26.

Rocco A, Fanali S. Analysis of phytosterols in extra-virgin olive oil by nano-liquid chromatography. *Journal of Chromatography A*. 2009;1216(43):7173–8.

Rodríguez-García C, Sánchez-Quesada C, Toledo E, et al. Naturally lignan-rich foods: A dietary tool for health promotion? *Molecules*. 2019;24(5):917.

Schwingshackl L, Hoffmann G. Monounsaturated fatty acids and risk of cardiovascular disease: synopsis of the evidence available from systematic reviews and meta-analyses. *Nutrients*. 2012;4(12):1989–2007.

Segura-Carretero A, Curiel JA. Current disease targets for oleocanthal as promising natural therapeutic agent. *International Journal of Molecular Science*. 2018;19(10):2899.

Serreli G, Deiana M. Biological relevance of extra virgin olive oil polyphenols metabolites. *Antioxidants* (Basel). 2018;7(12):170.

Simonsen NR, Fernandez-Crehuet Navajas J, Martin-Moreno JM, et al. Tissue stores of individual monounsaturated fatty acids and breast cancer: the EURAMIC study. European Community Multicenter Study on Antioxidants, Myocardial Infarction, and Breast Cancer. *American Journal of Clinical Nutrition*. 1998;68(1):134–41.

Sun W, Frost B, Liu J. Oleuropein, unexpected benefits! *Oncotarget*. 2017;8(11):17409.

Terés S, Barceló-Coblijn G, Benet M, et al. Oleic acid content is responsible for the reduction in blood pressure induced by olive oil. Proceedings of the National Academy of Science. 2008;105(37):13811–6.

Vallibhakara SA, Nakpalat K, Sophonsritsuk A, et al. Effect of vitamin E supplement on bone turnover markers in postmenopausal osteopenic women: a double-blind, randomized, placebo-controlled trial. *Nutrients*. 2021;13(12):4226.

Vilaplana-Pérez C, Auñón D, Garcia-Flores LA, et al. Hydroxytyrosol and potential uses in cardiovascular disease, cancer, and AIDS. *Frontiers in Nutrition*. 2014;1(18).

Visioli F, Bellomo G, Galli C. Free radical-scavenging properties of olive oil polyphenols. *Biochemical & Biophysical Research Communications*. 1998 Jun 9;247(1):60–4.

Wardhana, Surachmanto ES, Datau EA. The role of omega-3 fatty acids contained in olive oil on chronic inflammation. *Acta Med Indonesia*. 2011;43(2):138–43.

Waterman E, Lockwood B. Active components and clinical applications of olive oil. *Alternative Medicine Review*. 1007;12(4):331–42.

Yorulmaz HO, Konuskan DB. Antioxidant activity, sterol and fatty acid compositions of Turkish olive oils as an indicator of variety and ripening degree. *Journal of Food Science and Technology*. 2017;54(12):4067–77.

Chapter 3: The Heart-Healthy Oil

Aikawa M, Sugiyama S, Hill CC, et al. Lipid lowering reduces oxidative stress and endothelial cell activation in rabbit atheroma. *Circulation*. 2002;106(11):1390–6.

Al-Shudiefat AA, Ludke A, Malik A, et al. Olive oil protects against progression of heart failure by inhibiting remodeling of heart subsequent to myocardial infarction in rats. *Physiological Reports*. 2022;10:e15379.

Appel LJ, Moore TJ, Obarzanek E, et al. A clinical trial of the effects of dietary patterns on blood pressure. DASH Collaborative Research Group. *New England Journal of Medicine.* 1997;336:1117–24.

Bazal P, Gea A, de la Fuente-Arrillaga C, et al. Olive oil intake and risk of atrial fibrillation in the SUN cohort. *Nutrition, Metabolism, and Cardivascular Disease*. 2019;29(5):450–7.

Berrougui H, Ikhlef S, Khalil A. Extra virgin olive oil polyphenols promote cholesterol efflux and improve HDL functionality. *Evidence-Based Complementary and Alternative Medicine.* 2015;2015:208062.

Bukhari IA, Mohamed OY, Almotrefi AA, et al. Cardioprotective effect of olive oil against ischemic reperfusion-induced cardiac arrhythmia in isolated diabetic rat heart. *Cureus.* 2020;12(2):e7095.

Carnevale R, Pignatelli P, Nocella C, et al. Extra virgin olive oil blunt post-prandial oxidative stress via NOX2 down-regulation. *Atherosclerosis*. 2014;235(2):649–58.

Donat-Vargas C, Sandoval-Insausti H, Peñalvo JL, et al. Olive oil consumption is associated with a lower risk of cardiovascular disease and stroke. *Clinical Nutrition*. 2022;41(1):122–30.

Dokmanovic SK, Kolovrat K, Laskaj R, et al. Effect of extra virgin olive oil on biomarkers of inflammation in HIV-infected patients: a randomized, crossover, controlled clinical trial. *Medical Science Monitor*. 2015;21:2406–13.

Ferrara LA, Raimondi AS, d'Episcopo L, et al. Olive oil and reduced need for antihypertensive medications. *Archives of Internal Medicine.* 2000;160:837–42.

Guasch-Ferré M, Hu FB, Martínez-González MA. Olive oil intake and risk of cardiovascular disease and mortality in the PREDIMED Study. *BMC Medicine*. 2014;12:78.

Heart disease facts. Centers for Disease Control and Prevention. 2022. http://www.cdc.gov/heartdisease/facts.htm.

LDL and HDL Cholesterol and Triglycerides. Centers for Disease Control and Prevention. 2023.https://www.cdc.gov/cholesterol/ldl_hdl.htm.

Martínez-Gonzáez MA, Toledo E, Arós F, et al. Extra virgin olive oil consumption reduces risk of atrial fibrillation: The PREDIMED Trial. *Circulation*. 2014:130(1):18–26.

Menezes RCR, Peres, KK, Costa-Valle T, et al. Oral administration of oleuropein and olive leaf extract has cardioprotective effects in rodents: a systematic review. *Revista Portuguesa de Cardiologia*. 2022;41(2):167–75.

Moreno-Luna R, Munoz-Hernandez R, Miranda ML, et al. Olive oil polyphenols decrease blood pressure and improve endothelial function in young women with mild hypertension. *American Journal of Hypertension*. 2012;25:1299–304.

Njike VY, Ayettey R, Treu JA, et al. Post-prandial effects of a high poly-phenolic extra virgin olive oil on endothelial function in adults at risk of type 2 diabetes: A randomized controlled crossover trial. *International Journal of Cardiology*. 2021;330:171–6.

Ravnskov U, Diamond DM, Hama R. Lack of an association or an inverse association between low-density-lipoprotein cholesterol and mortality in the elderly: a systematic review. *BMJ Open*. 2016;6(6):e010401.

Ruiz-Canela M, Estruch R, Corella D, et al. Association of Mediterranean diet with peripheral artery disease. *JAMA*. 2014;311(4):415.

Sánchez-Quesada C, Toledo E, González-Mata G, et al. Relationship between olive oil consumption and ankle-brachial pressure index in a population at high cardiovascular risk. *Atherosclerosis.* 2020;314:48–57.

Sarapis K, Thomas CJ, Hoskin J, et al. The effect of high polyphenol extra virgin olive oil on blood pressure and arterial stiffness in healthy Australian adults: a randomized, controlled, cross-over study. *Nutrients.* 2020;12(8):2272.

Seidita A, Soresi M, Giannitrapani L, et al. The clinical impact of an extra virgin olive oil enriched Mediterranean diet on metabolic syndrome: lights and shadows of a nutraceutical approach. *Frontiers in Nutrition.* 2022;9:980429.

Sun W, Frost B, Liu J. Oleuropein, unexpected benefits! *Oncotarget.* 2017;9(11):17409.

What is atherosclerosis? National Heart, Lung, and Blood Institute. 2022. https://www.nhlbi.nih.gov/health/atherosclerosis.

Wongwarawipat T, Papgeorgiou N, Bertsias D, et al. Olive oil-related anti-inflammatory effects on atherosclerosis: potential clinical implications. *Endrocrine, Metabolic, and Immune Disorders Drug Targets.* 2018;18(1):51–62.

Chapter 4: EVOO's Anticancer Properties

Adekola K, Rosen ST, Shanmugam M. Glucose transporters in cancer metabolism. Current Opinions in Oncology. 2012;24(6):650–4.

Cancer data and statistics. Centers for Disease Control and Prevention. 2022. https://www.cdc.gov/cancer/dcpc/data/index.htm.

Chang K, Gunter MJ, Rauber F, et al. Ultra-processed food consumption, cancer risk and cancer mortality: a large-scale prospective analysis within the UK Biobank. *EClinicalMedicine.* 2023;56:101840.

Common types of cancer. National Cancer Institute. 2023. https://www.cancer.gov/types/common-cancers.

Donnem T, Reynolds A, Kuczynski E, et al. Non-angiogenic tumours and their influence on cancer biology. *Nature Reviews Cancer*. 2018;18:323–36.

Fadaka A, Ajiboye B Ojo O, et al. Biology of glucose metabolization in cancer cells. *Journal of Oncological Sciences*. 2917;3(2):45–51.

Fiolet T, Srour B, Sellem L, et al. Consumption of ultra-processed foods and cancer risk: results from NutriNet-Santé prospective cohort. BMJ. 2018;360:k322.

Foran JA, Carpenter DO, Hamilton MC, et al. Risk-based consumption advice for farmed Atlantic and wild Pacific salmon contaminated with dioxins and dioxin-like compounds. *Environmental Health Perspectives*. 2005;113(5):552–6.

Foran JA, Good DH, Carpenter DO, et al. Quantitative analysis of the benefits and risks of consuming farmed and wild salmon. *Journal of Nutrition*. 2005;135(11):2639–43.

Gil APR, Kodonis I, Ioannidis A, et al. The effect of dietary intervention with high-oleocanthal and oleacein olive oil in patients with early-stage chronic lymphocytic leukemia: a pilot randomized trial. *Frontiers in Oncology*. 2022;11:810249.

Goren L, Zhang G, Kaushik S, et al. (-)-Oleocanthal and (-)-oleocanthal-rich olive oils induce lysosomal membrane permeabilization in cancer cells. *PLoS One*. 2019;14(8):e02116024.

Hallmarks of cancer. World Cancer Research Fund International. https://www.wcrf.org/diet-activity-and-cancer/risk-factors/what-is-cancer-how-does-cancer-develop/.

Health risk of radon. U.S. Environmental Protection Agency. 2023. https://www.epa.gov/radon/health-risk-radon.

Hsu DJ, Gao J, Yamaguchi N, et al. Arginine limitation drives a directed codon-dependent DNA sequence evolution response in colorectal cancer cells. Science Advances. 2023;9(1):eade9120.

Jensen IJ, Eilertsen KE, Otnæs CHA, et al. An update on the content of fatty acids, dioxins, PCBs and heavy metals in farmed, escaped and wild Atlantic salmon (Salmo salar L.) in Norway. *Foods*. 2020;9(12):1901.

Jiang X, Wang J, Deng X, et al. The role of microenvironment in tumor angiogenesis. *Journal of Experimental & Clinical Cancer Research.* 2020;39:204.

Lieu EL, Nguyen T, Rhyne S, et al. Amino acids in cancer. *Experimental & Molecular Medicine.* 2020;52:15–30.

Lin BW, Gong CC, Song HF, et al. Effects of anthocyanins on the prevention and treatment of cancer. *British Journal of Pharmacology*. 2017;174(11):1226–43.

Lugano R, Ramachandran M, Dimberg A. Tumor angiogenesis: causes, consequences, challenges and opportunities. *Cellular and Molecular Life Sciences.* 2020;77(9):1745–70.

Markellos C, Ourailidou ME, Gavriatopoulou M, et al. Olive oil intake and cancer risk: A systematic review and meta-analysis. *PLoS One*. 2022;17(1):e0261649.

Martin-Moreno JM. The role of olive oil in lowering cancer risk: is this real gold or simply pinchbeck? *Journal of Epidemiology in Community Health*. 2000;54(10):726–7.

Nwosu ZC, Ward MH, Sajjakulnukit P, et al. Uridine-derived ribose fuels glucose-restricted pancreatic cancer. *Nature.* 2023;618:151–8.

Ozonoff D, Longneck MP. Epidemiologic approaches to assessing human cancer risk from consuming aquatic food resources from chemically contaminated water. *Environmental Health Perspectives.* 1991;90:141–6.

Pezzella F, Gatter K. Non-angiogenic tumours unveil a new chapter in cancer biology. *The Journal of Pathology.* 2015;235(3):384–96.

Protano C, Buomprisco G, Cammalleri V, et al. The carcinogenic effects of formaldehyde occupational exposure: A systematic review. *Cancers (Basel).* 2021;14(1):165.

Psaltopoulou T, Kosti RI, Haidopoulos D, et al. Olive oil intake is inversely related to cancer prevalence: a systematic review and meta-analysis of 13800 patients and 23340 controls in 19 observational studies. *Lipids in Health and Disease.* 2011;10:127.

Samson, K. Cancer cells 'addicted' to glucose could make promising target. *Oncology Times.* 2020;42(14):28–30,33.

Spoerri RV, Kuehni CE. Parental occupational exposure to benzene and the risk of childhood cancer: A census-based cohort study. *Environment International.* 2017;108:84–91.

Steenland K, Winquist A. PFAS and cancer, a scoping review of the epidemiologic evidence. *Environmental Research.* 2021;194:110690.

Taylor KW, Troester MA, Herring AH. Associations between personal care product use patterns and breast cancer risk among white and black women in the Sister Study. *Environmental Health Perspectives.* 2018;126(2):027011.

Types of cancer. Cancer Research UK. 2020. https://www.cancerresearchuk.org/what-is-cancer/how-cancer-starts/types-of-cancer.

van Vliet S, Provenza FD, Kronberg SL. Health-promoting phytonutrients are higher in grass-fed meat and milk. Frontiers in Sustainable Food Systems. 2021;4:2020.

Wang L, Du M, Wang K, et al. Association of ultra-processed food consumption with colorectal cancer risk among men and women: results from three prospective US cohort studies. *BMJ.* 2022;378:e068921.

What is cancer? Cancer Research UK. https://www.cancerresearchuk.org/about-cancer/what-is-cancer.

Xiaojiao Liu, Kezhen Lv. Cruciferous vegetables intake is inversely associated with risk of breast cancer: A meta-analysis. The Breast. 2013;22(3):309–13.

Zhang L, Rana I, Shaffer RM, et al. Exposure to glyphosate-based herbicides and risk for non-Hodgkin lymphoma: A meta-analysis and supporting evidence. Mutation Research/Reviews in Mutation Research. 2019;781:186–206.

Zhu L, Shu Y, Liu C, et al. Dietary glycemic index, glycemic load intake, and risk of lung cancer: A meta-analysis of observational studies. *Nutrition.* 2022;99–100:111676.

Chapter 5: EVOO's Brain Benefits

Ackerman S. Major Structures and Functions of the Brain. Discovering the Brain. Washington (DC): National Academies Press (US). 1992.

Alzheimer's disease facts & figures. The Alzheimer's Association. https://www.alz.org/alzheimers-dementia/facts-figures.

Alzheimer's: Drugs help manage symptoms. Mayo Clinic. 2022. https://www.mayoclinic.org/diseases-conditions/alzheimers-disease/in-depth/alzheimers/art-20048103.

Amel N, Wafa T, Samia D, et al. Extra virgin olive oil modulates brain docosahexaenoic acid level and oxidative damage caused by 2,4-Dichlorophenoxyacetic acid in rats. *Journal of Food Science and Technology.* 2016;53(3):1454–64.

Ballarini T, Melo van Lent D, Brunner J, et al on behalf of the DELCODE Study Group. Mediterranean diet, Alzheimer disease biomarkers, and brain atrophy in old age. *Neurology.* 2021;96(24):e2920–32.

Barisano G, Montagne A, Kisler K, et al. Blood-brain barrier link to human cognitive impairment and Alzheimer's Disease. *Nature Cardiovascular Research.* 2022;1(2):108–15.

Brothers HM, Gosztyla ML, Robinson SR. The physiological roles of amyloid-β peptide hint at new ways to treat Alzheimer's disease. *Frontiers in Aging Neuroscience.* 2018;10:118.

Chen KH, Reese EA, Kim HW. Disturbed neurotransmitter transporter expression in Alzheimer's disease brain. *Journal of Alzheimer's Disease.* 2011;26(4):755–66.

Farr SA, Price TO, Dominguez LJ, et al. Extra virgin olive oil improves learning and memory in SAMP8 mice. *Journal of Alzheimer's Disease.* 2012;28(1):81–92.

Gauthier S, Reisberg B, Zaudig M, et al. Mild cognitive impairment. The Lancet. 2006;367(9518):1262–70.

Gomes Gonçalves N, Vidal Ferreira N, Khandpur N, et al. Association between consumption of ultraprocessed foods and cognitive decline. *JAMA Neurology.* 2023;80(2):142–50.

Holland N, Robbins TW, Rowe JB. The role of noradrenaline in cognition and cognitive disorders. *Brain.* 2021;144(8):2243–56.

Jiang F, Mishra SR, Shrestha N, et al. Association between hearing aid use and all-cause and cause-specific dementia: an analysis of the UK Biobank cohort. *Lancet Public Health.* 2023;8(5):e329–38.

Kaddoumi A, Denney TS Jr, Deshpande G. Extra-virgin olive oil enhances the blood-brain barrier function in mild cognitive impairment: a randomized controlled trial. *Nutrients.* 2022;14(23):5102.

Kaur S, DasGupta G, Singh S. Altered neurochemistry in Alzheimer's disease: targeting neurotransmitter receptor mechanisms and therapeutic strategy. *Neurophysiology.* 2019;51:293–309.

Lauretti E, Luliano L, Praticò D. Extra-virgin olive oil ameliorates cognition and neuropathology of the 3xTg mice: role of autophagy. *Annals of Clinical and Translational Neurology.* 2017;4(8):564–74.

Lauretti E, Nenov M, Dincer O, et al. Extra virgin olive oil improves synaptic activity, short-term plasticity, memory, and neuropathology in a tauopathy model. *Aging Cell.* 2020;19(1):e13076.

Levakov G, Kaplan A, Meir AY, et al. The effect of weight loss following 18 months of lifestyle intervention on brain age assessed with resting-state functional connectivity. *eLife.* 2023;12:e83604.

Liu W, Li J, Yang M, et al. Chemical genetic activation of the cholinergic basal forebrain hippocampal circuit rescues memory loss in Alzheimer's disease. *Alzheimer's Research & Therapy.* 2022;14:53.

Murari G, Ri-Sheng Liang D, Ali A, et al. Prefrontal GABA levels correlate with memory in older adults at high risk for Alzheimer's disease. *Cerebral Cortex Communications.* 2020;1(1):tgaa022.

Peña-Bautista C, Baquero M, Vento M, et al. Free radicals in Alzheimer's disease: Lipid peroxidation biomarkers. *Clinica Chimica Acta*. 2019;491:85–90.

Petersen RC, Negash S. Mild Cognitive Impairment: An Overview. *CNS Spectrum.* 2008;13(1):45–53.

Pilozzi A, Carro C, Huang X. Roles of β-endorphin in stress, behavior, neuroinflammation, and brain energy metabolism. *International Journal of Molecular Science*. 2020;22(1):338.

Román GC, Jackson RE, Reis J, et al. Extra-virgin olive oil for potential prevention of Alzheimer's disease. *Reviews in Neurology.* 2019;175:705–23.

Sheffler ZM, Reddy V, Pillarisetty LS. Physiology, Neurotransmitters. [Updated 2023 May 1]. StatPearls [Internet]. Treasure Island (FL): StatPearls Publishing. 2023.

Snowden SG, Ebshiana AA, Hye A, et al. Neurotransmitter imbalance in the brain and Alzheimer's disease pathology. *Journal of Alzheimer's Disease*. 2019;72(1):35–43.

Solas M, Puerta E, Ramirez MJ. Treatment options in Alzheimer´s disease: The GABA story. *Current Pharmaceutical Design*. 2015;21(34):4960–71.

Tsolaki M, Lazarou E, Kozori M, et al. A randomized clinical trial of Greek high phenolic early harvest extra virgin olive oil in mild cognitive impairment: The MICOIL Pilot Study. *Journal of Alzheimer's Disease*. 2020;78(2):801–17.

Yang Z, Zou Y, Wang L. Neurotransmitters in prevention and treatment of Alzheimer's disease. *International Journal of Molecular Sciences*. 2023;24(4):3841.

Yuan TF, Li WG, Zhang C, et al. Targeting neuroplasticity in patients with neurodegenerative diseases using brain stimulation techniques. *Translational Neurodegeneration*. 2020;9:44.

Chapter 6: The Diabetes-Defying Power of EVOO

Alkhatib A, Tsang C, Tuomilehto J. Olive oil nutraceuticals in the prevention and management of diabetes: from molecules to lifestyle. *International Journal of Molecular Science*. 2018;19(7): 2024.

Beaudry KM, Devries MC. Nutritional strategies to combat type 2 diabetes in aging adults: the importance of protein. *Frontiers in Nutrition*. 2019;6:138.

Boulé NG, Kenny GP, Haddad E, et al. Meta-analysis of the effect of structured exercise training on cardiorespiratory fitness in Type 2 diabetes mellitus. *Diabetologia*. 2003;46(8):1071–81.

Carnevale R, Loffredo L, Del Ben M, et al. Extra virgin olive oil improves post-prandial glycemic and lipid profile in patients with impaired fasting glucose. *Clinical Nutrition*. 2017;36(3):782–7.

Common Side Effects of Diabetes Medication. London Diabetes Centre. https://londondiabetes.com/news-and-events/common-side-effects-of-diabetes-medication/.

Da Porto A, Brosolo G, Casarsa V, et al. The pivotal role of oleuropein in the anti-diabetic action of the Mediterranean diet: a concise review. *Pharmaceutics.* 2021;14(1):40.

Diabetes Prevention Program (DPP) Research Group. The Diabetes Prevention Program (DPP): description of lifestyle intervention. *Diabetes Care.* 2002;25(12):2165–71.

Diabetes UK. Diabetes in the UK 2010: Key statistics on diabetes. https://www.diabetes.org.uk/resources-s3/2017-11/diabetes_in_the_uk_2010.pdf.

Francois ME, Baldi JC, Manning PJ, et al. 'Exercise snacks' before meals: a novel strategy to improve glycaemic control in individuals with insulin resistance. *Diabetologia.* 2014;57:1437–45.

Jansson AK, Chan LX, Lubans DR, et al. Effect of resistance training on HbA1c in adults with type 2 diabetes mellitus and the moderating effect of changes in muscular strength: a systematic review and meta-analysis. *BMJ Open Diabetes Research & Care.* 2022;10(2):e002595.

Jayedi A, Soltani S, Zargar MS, et al. Central fatness and risk of all-cause mortality: systematic review and dose-response meta-analysis of 72 prospective cohort studies. *BMJ.* 2020;370:m3324.

Jurado-Ruiz E, Álvarez-Amor L, Varela LM, et al. Extra virgin olive oil diet intervention improves insulin resistance and islet performance in diet-induced diabetes in mice. *Scientific Reports.* 2019;9(1):11311.

Kirwan JP, Sacks J, Nieuwoudt S. The essential role of exercise in the management of type 2 diabetes. *Cleveland Clinic Journal of Medicine.* 2017;84(7 Suppl 1):S15–21.

Kouidrat Y, Pizzol D, Cosco T, et al. High prevalence of erectile dysfunction in diabetes: a systematic review and meta-analysis of 145 studies. *Diabetic Medicine.* 2017;34(9):1185–92.

Martínez-González MA, Sayón-Orea C, Bullón-Vela V, et al. Effect of olive oil consumption on cardiovascular disease, cancer, type

2 diabetes, and all-cause mortality: A systematic review and meta-analysis. *Clinical Nutrition*. 2022;41(12):2659–82.

Nakhanakhup C, Moungmee P, Appell HJ, et al. Regular physical exercise in patients with type II diabetes mellitus. *European Review of Aging and Physical Activity*. 2006;3:10.

National Diabetes Statistics Report. Centers for Disease Control and Prevention. 2022. https://www.cdc.gov/diabetes/data/statistics-report/index.html.

Qadir R, Sculthorpe NF, Todd T, et al. Effectiveness of resistance training and associated program characteristics in patients at risk for type 2 diabetes: a systematic review and meta-analysis. *Sports Medicine*. 2021;7:38.

Schwingshackl L, Lampousi AM, Portillo MP, et al. Olive oil in the prevention and management of type 2 diabetes mellitus: a systematic review and meta-analysis of cohort studies and intervention trials. *Nutrition & Diabetes*. 2017;7(4):e262.

Sonmez A, Yumuk V, Haymana C, et al. Impact of obesity on the metabolic control of type 2 diabetes: results of the Turkish Nationwide Survey of Glycemic and Other Metabolic Parameters of Patients with Diabetes Mellitus (TEMD Obesity Study). *Obesity Facts*. 2019;12(2):167–78.

Chapter 7: EVOO for Better Joint Health

Adami G, Viapiana O, Rossini M, et al. Association between environmental air pollution and rheumatoid arthritis flares. *Rheumatology* (Oxford). 2021;60(10):4591–7.

Almalty A, Hamed S, Tariah A, et al. The effect of topical application of extra virgin olive oil on alleviating knee pain in patients with knee osteoarthritis: a pilot study. *Indian Journal of Physiotherapy and Occupational Therapy*. 2013;7:6–11.

Arthritis. Centers for Disease Control and Prevention. 2021. https://www.cdc.gov/chronicdisease/resources/publications/factsheets/arthritis.htm.

Bayliss LE, Culliford D, Monk AP, et al. The effect of patient age at intervention on risk of implant revision after total replacement of the hip or knee: a population-based cohort study. *The Lancet*. 2017;389(10077):1424–30.

Beauchamp GK, Keast RS, Morel D, et al. Phytochemistry: ibuprofen-like activity in extra-virgin olive oil. *Nature.* 2005;437(7055):45–6.

Bhatt AP, Gunasekara DB, Speer J, et al. Nonsteroidal anti-inflammatory drug-induced leaky gut modeled using polarized monolayers of primary human intestinal epithelial cells. *ACS Infectious Disease.* 2018;4(1):46–52.

Casas R, Estruch R, Sacanella E. The protective effects of extra virgin olive oil on immune-mediated inflammatory responses. *Endocrine, Metabolic, & Immune Disorders Drug Targets.* 2018;18(1):23–35.

Chin KY, Pang KL. Therapeutic effects of olive and its derivatives on osteoarthritis: from bench to bedside. *Nutrients.* 2017;9(10):1060.

d'Angelo M, Brandolini L, Catanesi M, et al. Differential effects of nonsteroidal anti-inflammatory drugs in an in vitro model of human leaky gut. *Cells.* 2023;12:728.

De Vito R, Fiori F, Ferraroni M, et al. Olive oil and nuts in rheumatoid arthritis disease activity. *Nutrients*. 2023;15(4):963.

Diclofenac Topical (arthritis pain). Medline Plus. National Library of Medicine. 2021. https://medlineplus.gov/druginfo/meds/a611002.html.

Dolatkhah N, Toopchizadeh V, Barmaki S, et al. The effect of an anti-inflammatory in comparison with a low caloric diet on physical and mental health in overweight and obese women with knee osteoarthritis: a randomized clinical trial. *European Journal of Nutrition.* 2023;62(2):659–72.

Ferraz CR, Carvalho TT, Manchope MF, et al. Therapeutic potential of flavonoids in pain and inflammation: mechanisms of action, pre-clinical and clinical data, and pharmaceutical development. *Molecules.* 2020; 25(3):762.

Fransen M, Agallotis M, Nairn L, et al. Glucosamine and chondroitin for knee osteoarthritis: a double-blind randomised placebo-controlled clinical trial evaluating single and combination regimens. *Annals of the Rheumatic Diseases.* 2015;74:851–8.

Genel F, Kale M, Pavlovic N, et al. Health effects of a low-inflammatory diet in adults with arthritis: a systematic review and meta-analysis. *Journal of Nutritional Science.* 2020;9:e37. Hekmatpou D, Mortaji S, Rezaei M, et al. The effectiveness of olive oil in controlling morning inflammatory pain of phalanges and knees among women with rheumatoid arthritis: a randomized clinical trial. *Rehabilitation Nursing.* 2020;45(2):106–13.

Inacio MCS, Ake CF, Paxton EW, et al. Sex and risk of hip implant failure: assessing total hip arthroplasty outcomes in the United States. *JAMA Internal Medicine.* 2013;173(6):435–41.

Juneja P, Munjal A, Hubbard JB. Anatomy, Joints. [Updated 2023 Apr 1]. StatPearls [Internet]. Treasure Island (FL): StatPearls Publishing. 2023.

Kantor ED, Lampe JW, Navarro SL, et al. Associations between glucosamine and chondroitin supplement use and biomarkers of systemic inflammation. *Journal of Alternative and Complementary Medicine.* 2014;20(6):479–85.

Kenney C, Dick S, Lea J, et al. A systematic review of the causes of failure of Revision Total Hip Arthroplasty. *Journal of Orthopaedics.* 2019;16(5):393–5.

Kou H, Huang L, Jin M, et al. Effect of curcumin on rheumatoid arthritis: a systematic review and meta-analysis. *Frontiers in Immunology.* 2023;14:1121655.

Makris UE, Kohler MJ, Fraenkel L. Adverse effects of topical nonsteroidal anti-inflammatory drugs in older adults with osteoarthritis: a systematic literature review. *Journal of Rheumatology.* 2010;37(6):1236–43.

Messier SP, Mihalko SL, Beavers DP, et al. Effect of high-intensity strength training on knee pain and knee joint compressive forces among adults with knee osteoarthritis: the START randomized clinical trial. JAMA. 2021;325(7):646–57.

Musumeci G, Trovato FM, Pichler K, et al. Extra-virgin olive oil diet and mild physical activity prevent cartilage degeneration in an osteoarthritis model: an in vivo and in vitro study on lubricin expression. *Journal of Nutritional Biochemistry.* 2013;24(12):2064–75.

Osani MC, Bannuru RR. Efficacy and safety of duloxetine in osteoarthritis: a systematic review and meta-analysis. *Korean Journal of Internal Medicine.* 2019;34(5):966–73.

Osteoarthritis. National Institute of Arthritis and Musculoskeletal and Skin Diseases. 2019. https://www.niams.nih.gov/health-topics/osteoarthritis

Parkinson L, Keast R. Oleocanthal, a phenolic derived from virgin olive oil: a review of the beneficial effects on inflammatory disease. International Journal of Molecular Science. 2014;15(7):12323–34.

Perkins K, Sahy W, Beckett RD. Efficacy of curcuma for treatment of osteoarthritis. *Journal of Evidence-Based Complementary and Alternative Medicine.* 2017;22(1):156–65.

Pourhabibi-Zarandi F, Shojaei-Zarghani S, Rafraf M. Curcumin and rheumatoid arthritis: A systematic review of literature. *International Journal of Clinical Practice* 2021;75(10):e14280.

Rheumatoid Arthritis. Centers for Disease Control and Prevention. 2022. https://www.cdc.gov/arthritis/basics/rheumatoid-arthritis.html.

Rheumatoid Arthritis. National Institute of Arthritis and Musculoskeletal and Skin Diseases. https://www.niams.nih.gov/health-topics/rheumatoid-arthritis.

Rogers MAM, Aronoff DM. The influence of non-steroidal anti-inflammatory drugs on the gut microbiome. *Clinical Microbiology and Infection*. 2016;22(2):178.e1–e9.

Rosillo MÁ, Alarcón-de-la-Lastra C, Castejón ML, et al. Polyphenolic extract from extra virgin olive oil inhibits the inflammatory response in IL-1β-activated synovial fibroblasts. *British Journal of Nutrition*. 2019;121(1):55–62.

Sadeghi A, Zarrinjooiee G, Mousavi SN, et al. Effects of a Mediterranean diet compared with the low-fat diet on patients with knee osteoarthritis: a randomized feeding trial. *International Journal of Clinical Practice*. 2022;2022:7275192.

Total Joint Replacement. American Academy of Orthopaedic Surgeons. 2021. https://orthoinfo.aaos.org/en/treatment/total-joint-replacement/.

Van Ameyde M, Hodgden J. In patients with osteoarthritis, is curcumin, compared to placebo, effective in reducing pain? *Journal of the Oklahoma State Medical Association.* 2022;115(1):28–30.

Wang X, Liu D, Li D, et al. Combined treatment with glucosamine and chondroitin sulfate improves rheumatoid arthritis in rats by regulating the gut microbiota. *Nutrition & Metabolism* (London). 2023;20(1):22.

Wernecke C, Braun HJ, Dragoo JL. The effect of intra-articular corticosteroids on articular cartilage: a systematic review. *Orthopaedic Journal of Sports Medicine.* 2015;3(5):2325967115581163.

Zeng C, Wei J, Li H, et al. Effectiveness and safety of glucosamine, chondroitin, the two in combination, or celecoxib in the treatment of osteoarthritis of the knee. *Scientific Reports*. 2015;5:16827.

Zhu X, Sang L, Wu D, et al. Effectiveness and safety of glucosamine and chondroitin for the treatment of osteoarthritis: a meta-analysis of randomized controlled trials. *Journal of Orthopaedic Surgery and Research.* 2018;13(1):170.

Chapter 8: Enhance Your Immunity with EVOO

Almoselhy RIM. Extra virgin olive oil as nutritional therapeutic immune-enhancer. *International Journal of Family Studies, Food Science, and Nutrition Health.* 2021;4(2):26–45.

Autoimmune disorders. Medline Plus. National Library of Medicine. https://medlineplus.gov/ency/article/000816.htm.

Conde C, Escribano BM, Luque E, et al. Extra-virgin olive oil modifies the changes induced in non-nervous organs and tissues by experimental autoimmune encephalomyelitis models. *Nutrients.* 2019;11:2448.

D'Acquisto F. Affective immunology: where emotions and the immune response converge. Dialogues in Clinical Neuroscience. 2017;19(1):9–19.

Damiot A, Pinto AJ, Turner JE, et al. Immunological implications of physical inactivity among older adults during the COVID-19 pandemic. *Gerontology.* 2020;66(5):431–8.

Dhabhar FS. Effects of stress on immune function: the good, the bad, and the beautiful. *Immunology Research.* 2014;58(2-3):193–210.

Fernández del Río L, Gutiérrez-Casado E, Varela-López A, et al. Olive oil and the hallmarks of aging. *Molecules.* 2016;21(2):163.

Graham-Engeland JE, Sin NL, Smyth JM, et al. Negative and positive affect as predictors of inflammation: Timing matters. *Brain, Behavior and Immunology.* 2018;74:222–30.

Guasch-Ferré M, Li Y, Willett WC, et al. Consumption of olive oil and risk of total and cause-specific mortality among U.S. adults. *Journal of the American College of Cardiology.* 2022;79(2):101–12.

Huang J, Song P, Hang K, et al. Sleep deprivation disturbs immune surveillance and promotes the progression of hepatocellular carcinoma. *Frontiers in Immunology.* 2021;12:727959.

Krysin AP, Tolstikova TG, Dolgikh MP, et al. Synthesis and anti-inflammatory activity of tyrosol and its structural analogs. *Pharmaceutical Chemistry Journal.* 2019;52:907–11.

Lo Conte M, Antonini Cencicchio M, Ulaszewska M, et al. A diet enriched in omega-3 PUFA and inulin prevents type 1 diabetes by restoring gut barrier integrity and immune homeostasis in NOD mice. *Frontiers in Immunology.* 2023;13:1089987.

Martínez Leo EE, Peñafiel AM, Hernández Escalante VM, et al. Ultra-processed diet, systemic oxidative stress, and breach of immunologic tolerance. *Nutrition.* 2021;91–92:111419.

Magrone T, Spagnoletta A, Salvatore R, et al. Olive leaf extracts act as modulators of the human immune response. *Endocrinology, Metabolism, and Immune Disorders Drug Targets.* 2018;18(1):85–93.

Millman JF, Okamoto S, Teruya T, et al. Extra-virgin olive oil and the gut-brain axis: influence on gut microbiota, mucosal immunity, and cardiometabolic and cognitive health. *Nutrition Reviews.* 2021;79(12):1362–74.

Montoya T, Sánchez-Hidalgo M, Castejón ML, et al. Oleocanthal supplemented diet improves renal damage and endothelial dysfunction in pristane-induced systemic lupus erythematosus in mice. *Food Research International.* 2023;163:112140.

Muñoz-Garcia R, Sánchez-Hidalgo M, Montoya T, et al. Effects of oleacein, a new epinutraceutical bioproduct from extra virgin olive oil, in LPS-activated murine immune cells. *Pharmaceuticals.* 2022;15:1338.

Nagpal R, Shively CA, Register TC, et al. Gut microbiome-Mediterranean diet interactions in improving host health. *F1000Res.* 2019;8:699.

Obied HK, Prenzler PD, Omar SH, et al. Chapter Six–Pharmacology of Olive Biophenols, Editor(s): James C. Fishbein. *Advances in Molecular Toxicology.* 2012;6:195–242.

Omar SH. Oleuropein in olive and its pharmacological effects. *Scientia Pharmaceutica.* 2010;78(2):133–54.

Pojero F, Aiello A, Gervasi F, et al. Effects of oleuropein and hydroxytyrosol on inflammatory mediators: consequences on inflammaging. *International Journal of Molecular Science.* 2022;24(1):380.

Pourriyahi H, Yazdanpanah N, Saghazadeh A, et al. Loneliness: an immunometabolic syndrome. *International Journal of Environmental Research & Public Health.* 2021;18(22):12162.

Puertollano MA, Puertollano E, Alvarez de Cienfuegos G, et al. Olive oil, immune system and infection. *Nutr Hosp.* 2010;25(1):1–8.

Qiu F, Liang CL, Liu H, et al. Impacts of cigarette smoking on immune responsiveness: Up and down or upside down? *Oncotarget.* 2017;8(1):268–84.

Romundstad S, Svebak S, Holen A, et al. A 15-year follow-up study of sense of humor and causes of mortality: The Nord-Trøndelag Health Study. *Psychosomatic Medicine.* 2016;78(3):345–53.

Serreli G, Deiana M. Extra virgin olive oil polyphenols: modulation of cellular pathways related to oxidant species and inflammation in aging. *Cells.* 2020;9(2):478.

Shan C, Miao F. Immunomodulatory and antioxidant effects of hydroxytyrosol in cyclophosphamide-induced immunosuppressed broilers. *Poultry Science.* 2022;101(1):101516.

Silva S, Sepodes B, Rocha J, et al. Protective effects of hydroxytyrosol-supplemented refined olive oil in animal models of acute inflammation and rheumatoid arthritis. *Journal of Nutritional Biochemistry.* 2015;26(4):360–8.

Zabetakis I, Lrodan R, Norton C, et al. COVID-19: The inflammation link and the role of nutrition in potential mitigation. *Nutrients.* 2020;12:1466.

Chapter 9: How to Choose and Use Olive Oil

2022–2023 Grade and labeling standards for olive oil, refined olive oil, and olive-pomace oil. State of California Department of Food and Agriculture. https://www.cdfa.ca.gov/mkt/mkt/pdf/CA_Olive_Oil_Standards.pdf.

Allouche Y, Jiménez A, Gaforio JJ, et al. How heating affects extra virgin olive oil quality indexes and chemical composition. *Journal of Agriculture and Food Chemistry.* 2007;55(23):9646–54.

Almoselhy. Extra virgin olive oil as nutritional therapeutic immuno-enhancer. *International Journal of Family Studies, Food Science, and Nutrition Health.* 2021;4:26–45.

Aparicio-Soto M, Sánchez-Hidalgo M, Rosillo MÁ, et al. Extra virgin olive oil: a key functional food for prevention of immune-inflammatory diseases. *Food & Function.* 2016;7(11):4492–505.

California Olive Oil Council COOC Seal. https://cooc.com/certification-process/.

Casadei E, Valli E, Panni F, et al. Emerging trends in olive oil fraud and possible countermeasures. Food Control. 2021;124:107902.

Castañer O, Fitó M, López-Sabater MC, et al. The effect of olive oil polyphenols on antibodies against oxidized LDL. A randomized clinical trial. *Clinical Nutrition.* 2011;30(4):490–3.

De Alzaa F, Guillaume C, Ravetti L. Evaluation of Chemical and Physical Changes in Different Commercial Oils during Heating. Acta Scientific Nutritional Health. 2018;2(6):2–11.

Frankel EN, Mailer, RJ, Wang SC, et al. Evaluation of extra-virgin olive oil sold in California. 2011. http://vrisi36.com/wp-content/uploads/UCDavis-Report.pdf.

Gaforio JJ, Visioli F, Alarcón-de-la-Lastra C, et al. Virgin olive oil and health: summary of the III International Conference on Virgin Olive Oil and Health Consensus Report, JAEN (Spain) 2018. *Nutrients.* 2019;11(9):2039.

Guillén MD, Uriarte PS. Study by 1H NMR spectroscopy of the evolution of extra virgin olive oil composition submitted to frying temperature in an industrial fryer for a prolonged period of time. *Food Chemistry*. 2012;134(1):162–72.

Juneau M. The benefits of extra virgin olive oil on cardiovascular health. Prevention Watch. 2021. https://observatoireprevention.org/en/2021/03/16/the-benefits-of-extra-virgin-olive-oil-on-cardiovascular-health/.

Kishimoto N. Microwave heating induces oxidative degradation of extra virgin olive oil. *Food Science and Technology Research*. 2019;25(1):75–9.

Lazzerini C, Cifelli M, Domenici B. Pigments in extra-virgin olive oil: Authenticity and Quality. Products from Olive Tree. 2016.

Li X, Wang S, Flynn D. Refrigeration is not reliable in detecting olive oil adulteration. 2013. https://olivecenter.ucdavis.edu/media/files/refrigerationisnotreliablefinal.pdf.

Lozano-Castellón J, Fernando Rinaldi de Alvarenga J, Vallverdú-Queralt A, et al. Cooking with extra-virgin olive oil: A mixture of food components to prevent oxidation and degradation. *Trends in Food Science & Technology*. 2022;123:28–36.

Lozano-Castellón J, Vallverdú-Queralt A, Rinaldi de Alvarenga JF, et al. Domestic sautéing with EVOO: change in the phenolic profile. *Antioxidants*. 2020;9(1):77. NAOOA certified quality seal program. https://www.aboutoliveoil.org/certified-olive-oil-list.

Olive oil fraud rampant as demand skyrockets. National Public Radio. 2007. https://www.npr.org/2007/08/07/12571726/olive-oil-fraud-rampant-as-demand-skyrockets#.

Ramírez-Anaya J del P, Samaniego-Sánchez C, Castañeda-Saucedo MC, et al. Phenols and the antioxidant capacity of Mediterranean vegetables prepared with extra virgin olive oil using different domestic cooking techniques. *Food Chemistry*. 2015;188:430–8.

Saglam C, Tuna YT, Gecgel U, et al. Effects of olive harvesting methods on oil quality. APCBEE *Procedia*. 2014;8:334–42.

Sakar EH, Gharby S. Olive oil: extraction technology, chemical composition, and enrichment using natural additives. *Olive Cultivation*. 2022.

United States standards for grades of olive oil and olive-pomace oil. U.S. Department of Agriculture. 2010. https://www.ams.usda.gov/sites/default/files/media/Olive_Oil_and_Olive-Pomace_Oil_Standard%5B1%5D.pdf.

Weesepoel Y, Alewijn M, Wijtten M, et al. Detecting food fraud in extra virgin olive oil using a prototype portable hyphenated photonics sensor. *Journal of AOAC INTERNATIONAL*. 2021;104(1):7–15.

ABOUT THE AUTHOR

Terry Lemerond

Terry Lemerond is a natural health expert with over 55 years of experience helping people live healthier, happier lives. A much sought-after speaker and accomplished author, Terry shares his wealth of experience and knowledge in health and nutrition through his educational programs, including the Terry Talks Nutrition website TerryTalksNutrition.com—newsletters, pod- casts, webinars, and personal speaking engagements. Terry has also hosted Terry Talks Nutrition radio for the past 30 years. His books include:

Fight Disease With A Powerful Natural Seed

Nature's Disease Fighter: Andrographis

Type 2 Diabetes? Break Free Naturally, with Hintonia

Wake UP! Melatonin is For More Than Just Sleep

Relieve Pain without Side Effects

Trauma Comfrey, Nature's Healing Herb

Drug-Free Relief of Anxiety & Stress

Propolis, The Natural Way to Prevent and Heal Infection

The Wise Ginseng Choice for Restored Health: Red Ginseng

Polyphenol Power!

The Mediterranean Anti-Aging Secret to Vibrant Health

Outsmart Cancer with Powerful Natural Medicines

Reduce Fatty Liver with Herbal Medicines

Also available in paperback:

Seven Keys to Vibrant Health

Seven Keys to Unlimited Personal Achievement

50+ Natural Health Secrets Proven to Change Your Life

Discovering Your Best Health – How to Improve Your Health at Any Age

Terry continues to author and co-author books to educate everyone on the steps they can take to live a healthier, vibrant life.

His continual dedication, energy, and zeal are part of his ongoing mission—to help us all improve our health.

MORE ABOUT TTN PUBLISHING, LLC

Everyone has the same desire:
a vibrant, healthy life!

TTN Publishing exists to provide educational information anyone can use to understand how herbs and botanical medicines play a vital role in optimal health. From a stomachache to a life-threatening disease, even cancer, the plant kingdom has safe, effective phytonutrients and answers for healthy living.

Author and health pioneer Terry Lemerond brings his vast knowledge of plant medicines combined with cutting edge research from today's top scientists and doctors directly to consumers.

Each TTN Publishing, LLC book is crafted to provide the necessary basic information and recommendations for how botanicals can be used in practical ways to fight disease and improve the path to healthy living.

Education, information, scientific validation, and common sense are a part of every TTN Publishing endeavor. There are many books to come, so stay connected! With 80 percent of the world's population depending on plant medicines, you can join in the knowledge and wisdom available to meet your health goals.

WELCOME TO TTN PUBLISHING!

We'd love to hear from you!
info@ttnpublishing.com
www.TTNPublishing.com

Would you like to be one of the first to know the latest updates on Terry's books?

- Learn more about his background and new
- books
- See photos, videos, and the latest news
- Listen to Terry's radio show and podcasts, including archived programs on a multitude of subjects
- Sign up for a free weekly email newsletter and educational webinar notices

It's all available at TerryTalksNutrition.com

Don't forget to connect at:
www.facebook.com/TerryTalksNutrition

SHARE THIS EXCITING NEWS!

If you appreciated this book, please let others know.

- Pick up another copy and share with a friend
- Talk about it on social media
- Write a review on your blog or website
- Recommend this book to friends and family

Thank you for being a true health seeker!
TTN Publishing, LLC

ALSO BY TERRY LEMEROND AND AVAILABLE ON AMAZON

(Free in Kindle Unlimited and available in eBook and paperback)

Fight Disease with a Powerful, Natural Seed – The Wonders of French Grape Seed Extract
Prevent and Reverse: Cancer, Heart Disease, Diabetes, Alzheimer's & More
by Terry Lemerond and Ajay Goel M.S. Ph.D.
https://www.amazon.com/Fight-Disease-Powerful-Natural-Seed-ebook/dp/B08MB12PF9

Nature's Disease Fighter: Andrographis
Protection Against: Colds, flu, & upper respiratory infections, joint pain and arthritis, diabetes, heart disease, liver disease, cancer, and much more!
by Terry Lemerond and Alexander Panossian, Ph.D.
https://www.amazon.com/ANDROGRAPHIS-NATURAL-DISEASE-Terry- Lemerond-ebook/dp/B08T9XS846

Type 2 Diabetes? Break Free Naturally with Hintonia
by Terry Lemerond and Jacob Teitelbaum, M.D.
https://www.amazon.com/Type-Diabetes-Break-Naturally-Hintonia-ebook/dp/B08ZT3TVP4

Relieve Pain Without Side Effects: You Can Be Pain-free, Naturally!
by Terry Lemerond and Jan McBarron M.D.
https://www.amazon.com/Relieve-Pain-Without-Side-Effects-ebook/dp/B091QCJW51

Wake UP! Melatonin is For More Than Just Sleep
The answer to aging, immune health, cancer, and much more!
by Terry Lemerond and a forward by Jacob Teitelbaum, M.D
https://www.amazon.com/Wake-Melatonin-More-Than-Sleep-ebook/dp/B092KZHR88

Trauma Comfrey, Nature's Healing Herb
Wounds, Sports Injuries, Sprains & Strains, Bruises, Back & Joint Pain and More
by Terry Lemerond and Holly Lucille, ND, RN
https://www.amazon.com/Trauma-Comfrey-Natures-Healing- Herb-ebook/dp/B09JWRMCLJ

Drug-Free Relief of Anxiety & Stress
Nature's Answer to Live Without Anxiety, Stress, Stress-induced Diseases
by Terry Lemerond and Dr. Lynn Wagner
https://www.amazon.com/Drug-Free-Relief-Anxiety-Stress-Stress-Induced-ebook/dp/B09JWVQV18

Propolis The Natural Way to Prevent and Heal Infection: Fights Infection Including: Bacterial, Viral, Fungal, Parasitic, and More
by Terry Lemerond
https://www.amazon.com/Propolis-Natural-Prevent-Heal-Infection/dp/1952507227

Restore Your Health with the Wise Ginseng Choice
by Terry Lemerond and Jacob Teitelbaum MD

Polyphenol Power! Polyphenols in fruit and vegetables to prevent and cure: Heart Disease, Cancer, Type 2 Diabetes, Alzheimer's and more!
by Terry Lemerond
https://www.amazon.com/POLYPHENOL-POWER-Polyphenols-vegetables-Alzheimers-ebook/dp/B0B6Q7GS9F

Outsmart Cancer with Powerful Natural Medicines
The Five Alternative Solutions to Prevent and Treat Cancer
by Terry Lemerond and Ajay Goel, Ph.D., AGAF
https://www.amazon.com/Outsmart-Cancer-POWERFUL-NATURAL-MEDICINES-ebook/dp/B0C6X7NQ5Q

The Mediterranean Anti-Aging Secret to Vibrant Health.

Greek Mountain Tea is the Ancient Secret to: Improved Mental Clarity. Reduced Anxiety. Strong Immunity. Bone Density. Preventing Alzheimer's Disease

by Terry Lemerond

https://www.amazon.com/MEDITERRANEAN-ANTI-AGING-SECRET-VIBRANT-HEALTH-ebook/dp/B0C5KFXSF6

Reduce Fatty Liver Disease with HERBAL MEDICINES

by Terry Lemerond and Dr. Lexi Loch

https://www.amazon.com/Reduce-Fatty-Disease-HERBAL-MEDICINES-ebook/dp/B0CCBT5F8T

Additional paperback books available on Amazon:

Terry Talks Nutrition 50+ Natural Health Secrets Proven to Change Your Life

Discovering Your Best Health

How To Improve Your Health at Any Age

Seven Keys to Vibrant Health

Seven Keys to Unlimited Personal Achievement

Made in United States
North Haven, CT
04 November 2026

21768986R00106